Cortisone

Cortisone

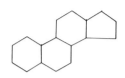

Edward C. Kendall

Illustrated with photographs

Charles Scribner's Sons · New York

TO MY WIFE, MY SON HUGH, MY DAUGHTER ELIZABETH,
AND TO THE MEMORY OF MY SONS ROY AND NORMAN

Contents

Illustrations

Cortisone

One

I Choose Chemistry

MY FOREBEARS CAME from England and Scotland to the New England colonies, the first of them in 1636, and gradually moved to western Massachusetts and Connecticut. At least one crossed the Hudson River: Robert Roy (1792-1832) was pastor of the Old Tennent Church in Tennent, New Jersey.

My paternal grandfather, Calvin Hemingway Kendall (1817-1904), I remember as a tall serious-looking man with long thick white hair brushed straight back from a high forehead. He also wore a white beard but his upper lip was not hidden beneath a mustache. He was deacon in the Congregational Church in Ridgefield, Connecticut, where he lived; when you watched him serve bread and wine on communion Sunday you understood why he was held in high esteem as a pillar of the church and a respected elder of the community. For him and his family Sunday was the Lord's day, and diversions of any kind, such as skating in the winter or a picnic in the summer, were not even temptations—they were simply excluded from consideration.

Grandfather did have one indulgence, however. Though he did not use tobacco in any form, he enjoyed the taste of quinine. At intervals throughout the day he would reach into his coat pocket for a miniature bottle of finely crystalline quinine, open a small pocket knife, withdraw a few crystals of the bitter alkaloid on the knife

1

blade, and place them on his tongue. I never asked him why and he never explained.

Calvin H. Kendall married Jane Ann Roy in 1846. They had a family of three boys, John, Robert, and George. The children grew to manhood in the puritanical atmosphere of the Kendall home, and they in turn carried on the precepts they learned as children. John graduated with high honors from a medical school and became a physician in Norfolk, Connecticut. Robert graduated from a Presbyterian seminary and was pastor of a church in Weymouth, Massachusetts, and George Stanley Kendall, my father, chose dentistry for a vocation. My father had a retiring disposition and could not have been happy as a clergyman. He was a patient, meticulous craftsman and had a wide reputation in his chosen field. His father had also been a dentist, but dentistry in the middle decades of the nineteenth century was not the profession into which it was developed after 1900.

After graduation from the New York School of Dentistry my father married Eva Frances Abbott. They made their home in South Norwalk, Connecticut, where their three children were born: Florence R. Kendall, March 7, 1877; Ruth Dodge Kendall, May 24, 1884; and Edward C. Kendall, March 8, 1886.

My maternal grandparents died while I was quite young, but I do recall one visit in their home. It was memorable because of all the trouble made by a motorman on the local trolley about a small boy who suddenly ran across the street in front of his car. I am sure that I could have beaten that record for running across the street if we had visited there again.

Puritanical beliefs must also have influenced my mother's upbringing. She was an able and active worker in the Congregational Church, and she concurred with Father in regard to the conduct of family life. From the time we were small children, all members of the Kendall family ate breakfast, lunch, and dinner together. At breakfast we did not appear in pajamas, sweaters, and slippers, or nightgowns, kimonos, and night caps. We were fully clothed and shod, with faces washed, teeth brushed, and hair combed or braided. Father always recited a blessing at meals, but we did not have daily family worship. On Sunday evenings the family assembled in the

2

living room; Father read a chapter or so from the Bible; we all sang a short hymn and knelt in front of our chairs while Father offered a prayer. In addition, we were taught to say our prayers each night, on our knees.

The horrors of Dante's *Divine Comedy* and the bliss of heavenly existence were accepted by me as facts not to be questioned. But such a well-arranged and beautiful world could not last for many years. It was somewhat shaken but not crushed by two incidents. Of course I knew that it was wrong and unforgivable to swear but one day I was alone, standing near a telephone pole, when I decided to see what would happen if I did swear. I said, "God damn," not to myself but out loud. I would not have been surprised if a bolt of lightning had smashed that pole into fine splinters. When nothing at all happened I began to wonder how much further I could go down forbidden ways and get away with it.

The second incident was even more provocative. Mother had taken me to stay a few days with my paternal grandparents in Ridgefield. Grandfather and I were seated on the front porch. It was obvious that he had something on his mind when he turned to me and said, "Isn't it funny, here we are today but we don't know where we will be tomorrow."

That remark has remained with me for more than seven decades. It would be interesting to compare my thoughts as each decade was passed, but no record was made. My immediate reaction was one of surprise and shock. Surprise, because I knew where I would be, and I thought that anyone as old as Grandfather surely would know where he would be. I was shocked because, if Grandfather really did not know, then who, in all the world, could tell me? I began to wonder, to question.

In 1890 my parents built a new home on a broad plateau northwest of the city. The address was 51 Elmwood Avenue, and the property was separated from the outer edge of town by one block. Beyond that there were only woods and farms.

My boyhood was spent in the new home. The house had four rooms on the first and second floors, and one room was finished with lath and plaster walls in the attic. This was for the maid. We always had a maid who "slept in" at our house. Many of these maids were from

Hungary. For the chance to learn English and the American way of life they were glad to work for room and board plus seven or eight dollars a month.

Most of the large attic was left unfinished, and there in front of a window that looked out toward the southwest I made a workbench that allowed me to make "things." Telegraph instruments, induction coils, electromagnets, and as time passed I worked long and hard to devise a telephone circuit such that when I removed a telephone receiver from its hook in my home a bell would ring in the second house from ours. It would continue to ring until my friend Freeman Light removed the receiver at his end. The bell then stopped ringing and two-way conversation could be carried on.

The attic workshop acquired new importance when I was able to make over an old sewing machine into a lathe that could drill a hole in a piece of sheet brass or steel. This modification of the sewing machine required a certain amount of work in a machine shop and I found unanticipated pleasure in Miller's Machine Shop on Water Street. Friday afternoon after school and on Saturday I passed many a happy hour watching the metal strips curl off a lathe or planing machine.

Another favorite pastime was to watch the work at the Norwalk Cast Iron Foundry. The blast furnace with its charge of molten iron was tapped in the afternoon, and the white-hot metal was poured into a large bucket that was transported by an overhead electric crane. The liquid cast iron was then tipped out of the bucket into the many molds that had been prepared. These operations were accompanied by showers of sparks, rumbling of motors, clanking of chains, some shouting and running around. It was a fascinating show and as I became recognized by the workmen they allowed certain privileges not open to the occasional visitor.

When I was in the eighth grade, the teacher gave cards to all the pupils and asked them to write their names and what they intended to do when they grew up. My answer was: I want to be a philosopher. I do not know whether I spelled the word correctly and I doubt if I could have given its dictionary definition. What I meant was that I was very much interested in mechanical things and natural phenomena and wanted to know more about what "made the wheels go round."

4

For recreation Long Island Sound lay close at hand. The family belonged to a shore resort club, The Knob. Most of the summer vacations were spent in and on the water.

Another source of pleasure was a suspension bridge between two tall Norway pine trees in our back yard. The trees were about thirty feet apart and more than thirty feet tall. The bridge was about fifteen feet off the ground and was only one foot wide, but it was enough for two young boys to sit on or cross over from one tree to the other. Lunch never tasted so good as it did when we pulled it up to the bridge with a rope.

In 1901 I entered the South Norwalk High School and came under the guidance of Miss Charlotte Lamont. My sister Florence had been a pupil of Miss Lamont and since that time she had been a close friend of the family. She taught geometry and Latin and she made both subjects clear and logical. Ever since high school days I have been grateful for her leadership, for she laid the foundation of my scholastic career.

The course of my life throughout high school was determined by the progress in the courtship of my sister Florence. When she entered the South Norwalk High School she met Mark W. Norman. He and his brother Hugart lived with their uncle, Mark Wilbur, in Darien, Connecticut. From first sight Florence and Mark fell in love with each other, and from that day for the rest of their lives that love remained mutual and constant.

Physically, Mark was a powerfully built man. He neither smoked nor drank; he excelled as an athlete and was fullback on a winning football team of Columbia University. At the same time he maintained a good scholastic record and graduated in the class of 1900. Mark entered his uncle's law office in New York City and married my sister in June 1902.

The years that I attended high school were strongly influenced by the life of Mark W. Norman. He was my friend, my mentor, and my idol. When the time came to select where I should go to college the matter was settled promptly. Columbia University was the alma mater of Mark; I too chose Columbia.

The high school at South Norwalk had only a three-year course and when I picked Columbia for college it seemed best to attend a high school that covered four years of preparatory work. The near-

5

est high school was in Stamford, a city only eight miles from South Norwalk.

It required only a short time to decide that I should transfer to that institution. This I did in September 1903.

Before I went to the Stamford High School there was no doubt in my mind that I would choose some part of the field of physics for my vocation, but during the year I was introduced to the magical world of chemistry. It was fortunate for me that while I was there the faculty was outstanding. The teacher of chemistry had a Ph. D. from Yale University. The course that he taught was merely an introduction to chemistry but to me it was most interesting. I could appreciate the challenge that arose from a study of experiments carried out in the laboratory. I realized how rewarding it would be to discover how to manufacture new products or how to improve ways to make familiar compounds. These thoughts were new to me; they enlarged my horizon. I requested Columbia University to send a catalogue that described courses in chemistry, and after careful consideration I decided to make chemistry my vocation.

This decision was confirmed and strengthened from a wholly unanticipated source. When my sister Florence and Mark were married they started housekeeping in the home of Mark's uncle, Mr. Wilbur. It was about three miles between our house and the new home in Darien and I was a frequent visitor, via my bicycle. Mr. Wilbur was in the seventh decade of life and if the newlyweds were away for an evening I would ride over to spend the hours with the retired attorney. Mr. Wilbur had an endless stock of stories, both of personal experiences and of events, and he told them well.

On one of these occasions, Uncle Mark, as we all called him, told the adventurous story of a chemist in the paper industry. The problem that confronted him was to treat writing paper so that ink would not run and become blurred. The struggles of this man fascinated me the more because I knew it was a true story. The chemist was Uncle Mark's own brother, George Wilbur.

For some years he worked alone in a laboratory in his home. His wife had faith in the venture, and, as their reserve of money disappeared, she did the only work she could—sewing, washing, and ironing. After severe hardships he devised the essential solution and was able to treat the writing paper of a large industrial company. The agreement was that he would prepare the solution for use, but the ingredients and method of preparation would remain his secret. Since the paper company required his service, he was able to secure a high financial return and soon became affluent. The paper company tried very hard to discover his secret but he worked behind locked doors and rejected offers of assistance. He knew full well that as soon as the assistant deciphered his secret formula, his own service no longer would be needed.

It was a story of research, dogged persistence, intrigue, and a gamble with the future. To a young man the chance to turn near defeat into success outweighed other aspects and to me it afforded a strong motivation.

Uncle Mark had another spine-chilling story about a young man —not himself—who walked from New York to Brooklyn on the "cat-walk" of the Brooklyn Bridge when that structure was under construction in 1884. The "catwalk" is used by workmen before the floor of the bridge is laid. It is hung just below the cables that support the suspension bridge. It rises up to the top of the first tower, then goes down to the low point in the middle of the bridge, rises again to the top of the second tower, and descends to the ground. That story remained in my mind and later in this book I shall refer to it again.

The school year at Stamford passed quickly. I enjoyed athletics but I was too lightweight for the football team and commuting interfered with the required practice and training of basketball and other sports. However, I tried to keep in good physical condition. Weather permitting, occasionally I walked home the eight miles, and a group of my classmates walked with me from Stamford to New York City —about twenty-five miles.

College entrance examinations came in the spring. Although I had had only three years of high school, I took these in the spring of 1904. They were held in the gymnasium at Columbia and lasted for three long hours for each one. The labored grind of trolley cars climbing the long hill on Broadway and on Amsterdam Avenue was the only sound to break the silence of those fateful hours. I passed all of them and was accepted as a freshman to enter Columbia in September 1904.

Two

Columbia University

AT THE BEGINNING of my freshman year at Columbia I joined the Sigma Alpha Epsilon fraternity. Each fraternity on the campus strove to have its members excel in athletics or other activities that involved competition. For me football was out of consideration, but I entered elimination trials to represent the class of 1908 in the rugged and noble sport known as "cane spree." This contest between representatives of the freshman and sophomore classes was an annual event, held during the winter months. It comes closer to wrestling than to any other sport.

My next enlistment in the sports area was rowing. Beginning in January candidates for the crew began "rowing" on machines in the gymnasium. The oarsmen sat on a seat that moved back and forward on a track with each stroke. The resistance of the "oar" was determined by the tension of a band around a drum. A daily "row" for thirty minutes developed the muscles in preparation for the day we would go out on the water. This we did on the Harlem River during the latter half of March.

My experience as bow oar in a four-man shell culminated in an inter-fraternity race on the Hudson River. The bow man steers the shell and thereby has responsibility for the psychological response of the crew; if the shell is not kept on a straight course the crew will not give their utmost. Several crews were entered but the two crews that rowed stroke for stroke side by side for the entire course were Alpha Delta Phi and S.A.E. We won by a narrow margin. An ornate plaque bearing the names of the crew was presented to our fraternity and was given a place of honor on the wall of the living room in the fraternity house. In addition each member of the crew was given a bronze medal.

In the field of sports those who win first, second, and third place are rewarded with medals of gold, silver, and bronze respectively. We were given bronze medals only because the sponsors of the contest could not afford more expensive ones. But we had won and we were entitled to medals of the purest gold. Under these circumstances I believed it was perfectly ethical to convert my bronze medal into a gold one—at least on the outside. For one who had recourse to electroplating this was no problem at all. I gold-plated the bronze medal. This enhanced its beauty and also established its authenticity as a gold medal for first place in a hard-fought race.

Many years later, in 1952, when I was awarded the prestigious Kober Medal by the Association of American Physicians, Dr. Philip S. Hench of the Mayo Clinic, who was to make the presentation, asked me for some anecdotes of my youth. I told him the story of the crew race and the gold-plated medal. The story pleased him. He included it in his remarks and admonished me not to tinker with the Kober Medal. This amused the audience and made a happy ending for Dr. Hench, but there was one more smile known only to myself. On the obverse side of the medal was the statement "Awarded to Edward C. Kendall M.D." I am a member of the Association of American Physicians but I do not have the M.D. degree. And so the goldsmith, but not I, did have to tinker with the Kober Medal.

The change from my sheltered and restricted life at home to the give and take in a fraternity house in New York City was an important chapter in my life. I could not suddenly forget that Sunday was included in each week to permit mankind to withdraw from the world of men, to go to church, to think and read about religion.

Two members of my fraternity were of special help. One, Stuart Myers, was the son of the assistant pastor of the Marble Collegiate Church in New York City. I joined that church and was a faithful member of the congregation. Frequently I was invited for

Sunday dinner at the Myers home. The other fraternity brother was Walter Phelps Hall, who is described in Chapter 3; here I want to record one of his remarks that reveals his sense of values. He used to say that my religious beliefs did not stop me from departing the straight and narrow path—such as in playing cards, especially on Sunday—but they did prevent me from enjoying the infraction. During the four years of college the tight bonds of religious beliefs and observances of childhood days were somewhat loosened but by no means broken. I must have been a poor "mixer," but I found diversion and fascination in the laboratory.

I was fortunate in being able to study with Professors Frederick Chandler, Marston T. Bogart, Henry C. Sherman, and their colleagues. Their names need no praise from me, for they have long since passed into the recorded history of Columbia University. These men fulfilled my desire to know something of the laws of chemistry. They guided my steps and taught me that there is no substitute for knowledge. In the search for knowledge there is no substitute for truth.

After my graduation in 1908 I was appointed a laboratory instructor for the summer school session of six weeks. I believe my services were appreciated. One young lady gave me a poem she had written about the "Ken do all man." The laboratory where I spent the day occupied the entire west section of the second floor of Havemeyer Hall. This chemistry building was an architectural triumph of high ceilings, wide windows, and massive, broad, stone window sills. The window in the center of the west wall was at least six feet wide and the sill was not less than eighteen inches deep. The sill had a slight slope to shed rain water but it was almost flat.

I lived at home that summer and commuted to New York. As I had to take an early morning train, by noon I was hungry and tired. Diligent search on my part failed to discover any place on that floor where I could lie down. I looked at that wide window and found an answer.

I tried the sill for length and found that I could lie flat on my back without bending my knees. With a telephone book for a pillow and a handkerchief over my eyes I could sleep fifteen or twenty minutes, and awake refreshed and ready for the afternoon. Except in inclement weather this became a daily routine.

In the fall of 1908 I began graduate work in chemistry at Columbia. During the next spring vacation an opportunity arose to realize a daydream long cherished.

I had thought many times of the trip via the catwalk of the Brooklyn Bridge from New York to Brooklyn, and in the spring of 1909 my interest was renewed by the construction of another suspension bridge across the East River—the Manhattan Bridge. One day at the fraternity house I interested three other Columbia students in seeing whether we could repeat the feat that had been achieved twenty-seven years earlier. We went down to the New York end of the new bridge and found the superintendent of construction in his small office. We asked permission to go to Brooklyn by way of the catwalk. We promptly received an unqualified no, but the construction chief proved to be a good sport and after we said we would sign a statement that would relieve the company of all responsibility, financial or otherwise, his no was changed to yes. The catwalk was not made like a paved roadway. It was nothing more than pieces of 2-by-4 timber laid about an inch apart crossways. There was nothing but a rope on each side. It was waist high. There were two reasons for the catwalk. It provided transportation for men and material, and after all the single strands of wire in the cable were in place the catwalk was used to coat the wire cables with thick vaseline-like material and then to install the cover of the cable to hold the grease in place and exclude rain water.

The grease was a surprise to all of us. There was a thick smear of it on every square inch of the walk all the way to Brooklyn and it made the walk as slippery as ice. It did not seem slippery at first but as the catwalk became more and more steep the footing became less and less certain, and the distance down to the ground increased with each step. When we were near the top of the first tower the catwalk seemed to ascend like a ladder but instead of rungs for our feet the endless greasy 2-by-4 timbers stretched as far as we could see. I wondered whether the construction superintendent really thought we would go on.

The view from the top of the first tower was superb and was ample reward for the effort expended. I congratulated the three other climbers but when I looked at the shortest member I was startled. He was as white as a sheet and his actions showed that he was not comfortable. He was scared—very much so. It would have been impossible to carry him back and we could not leave him there alone. We rested at the top of the tower and gave each other advice and moral support. After a while we were all able to proceed, but now the situation was reversed—we were going down a very steep slope on a slippery wooden catwalk. There was nothing ahead but more of the same.

The view from the top of the second tower was magnificent but psychologically there was a vast difference from that of the first tower. Now we looked down on the end of the long journey. We were almost in Brooklyn. The rest at the top of the second tower was short and the end of the excursion came quickly. We were the first nonprofessional pedestrians to cross over the East River on the new Manhattan Bridge. I was happy to have matched Uncle Mark's story about the Brooklyn Bridge.

In 1909 Dr. Samuel Goldschmidt established a fellowship in the department of chemistry at Columbia University. I was the first recipient and had the good fortune to continue my graduate work at Columbia under the guidance of Professor H. C. Sherman. At that time Professor Sherman was interested in the action of enzymes—in particular the conversion of starch into maltose by pancreatic amylase.

Sixty years ago a few enzymes were articles of commerce, but their chemical nature was not known and the way an enzyme produced a chemical reaction was a matter of speculation. I too was interested in enzymes, and when Dr. Sherman asked whether I would like to work in this field for my Ph.D. thesis I said I would. He suggested that I try to devise a method to determine the potency of different samples of pancreatic amylase. That field of research had hitherto yielded few of its secrets. I hoped to find something of lasting value.

During the first months of the college year 1909–1910 I became adept with the techniques required for the research and also reviewed the literature on the action of enzymes. Work in the laboratory convinced me that the determination of maltose through the use of Fehling's Method was accurate and consistent; that is, a series of identical analyses with a single sample of the sugar would all agree within a small margin of error. However, such a statement could not be made concerning the amount of starch that was converted to maltose through the action of pancreatic amylase. The same amounts of two different preparations of amylase gave quite different results. Still more confusing, if the weight of a single sample of amylase was doubled or tripled, it did not follow that the sugar formed from starch during a constant period of time was twice or three times the first amount. It became evident that the activity of the enzyme depended on the conditions that were present in each separate flask when the experiment was carried out.

For me this observation was an anticlimax to my eager expectations. Ominous questions came to mind. Was such a conclusion worthy of a Ph.D. degree? Did I want to continue this type of research? These thoughts did not persist, nor did they affect my efforts to determine the cause for the variable behavior of pancreatic amylase. But time was precious; only three months remained and I had not started to write the all-important thesis.

A sober, careful review of the months of work indicated that the variable behavior of the enzyme might be caused by slight variations in the presence of inorganic material, such as salt. Graduate students in the department of chemistry washed their own glassware with ordinary cold tap water. Distilled water was not used even to rinse the tap water off the glass. It occurred to me to investigate the effect of traces of sodium chloride on the conversion of starch to maltose by pancreatic amylase. Salt was added to one of several flasks. The result was truly astonishing. The sample of pancreatin, which in previous experiments had a low potency, converted starch to maltose at a rate beyond all expectation. It was immediately evident that the enzymic activity of pancreatin was dependent on the presence of certain salts in the solution.

A door had been opened. A method to study the reactivity of pancreatin was speedily devised, and although the time available was short I was able to write a thesis for the Ph.D. degree that included not only experimental work carried out in the laboratory but also the derivations of differential and integral equations that expressed the rate of formation and the amount of maltose that would be produced from starch in any given period of time.

After submitting a thesis based on original work the candidate for the Ph.D. degree in chemistry was required to "defend the thesis" before a small group of professors in the department and then to meet with at least seven members for the final comprehensive oral examination. This sometimes lasted three hours. During my oral examination an incident occurred the relevance of which will be apparent later. When Professor Samuel Tucker was invited to examine me on electro-chemistry, he said he would not examine me on that subject, but he wondered whether I knew anything about an item that recently had come to his attention. The question concerned the presence of iodine in the thyroid gland, and I was obliged to answer it with an unqualified no. I did not know that iodine was a normal constituent of the thyroid gland. He did not question me further and the examination was brought to a close. A few days later, I was awarded my Ph.D. degree.

It was good to be alive. I was able to say to Professor Sherman, "This is the answer to your assignment of last September." The haunting question of whether I wanted to continue to work in the creative field of research in organic chemistry was banished. I was anxious to meet the next challenge.

Three

Parke Davis and St. Luke's Hospital

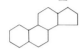

ON COMMENCEMENT DAY in June 1910 I sent a telegram to the director of the chemical laboratory at Parke Davis and Co. in Detroit, Michigan, asking for an interview. It was granted and at Detroit I met Dr. Jones. Dr. Jones did not say what project would be assigned to me and he did not discuss what facilities were available. However, he did agree that I could report for work on September 1, 1910. My salary would be $1350 a year.

On the appointed day I arrived at the company's manufacturing plant on East Jefferson Avenue, where I had a conference with Dr. Jones on the work I was to do. It was to isolate the active agent—that is, the hormone—of the thyroid gland. Whether Dr. Jones detected a smile on my face I do not know; I was thinking of Dr. Tucker's question.

I shall always be grateful to Dr. Jones for one thing: he introduced me to the thyroid gland. Otherwise, experience in the chemical laboratory of Parke Davis was a disappointment. I was looking for an institution where research in chemistry was carried on. What I found in my new position was far removed from what I anticipated. In 1910 Parke Davis and Co. was one of the leading pharmaceutical manufacturing firms in the United States, a position it held because of rigid control through chemical analysis of all products bought and sold. For this work the company had

17

installed a "control laboratory." I was given a small room in this laboratory. Supplies of chemicals and apparatus came through the administrator. Of all the chemists in the "control laboratory," I was the only one with a Ph.D. and the only one engaged in research.

Two aspects of the job greatly annoyed me. One was the edict that all those who worked in the laboratory were obliged to "punch" in and out on the time clock. After working eighteen hours a day for some weeks to finish my thesis I could not accept the thought that my value to the company could be determined by the hours spent in the building.

The second aspect was psychological. When I looked at my fellow workers and realized the stereotyped life that was their lot I resented the depressing atmosphere and the absence of any professional stimulation, such as lectures from visiting scientists or organized seminars or travelogues. I could not contemplate the future without a strong feeling of claustrophobia and frustration.

At the end of December I told Dr. Jones about the time clock and my dread of the future if the past four months were any indication of it. He insisted that I continue to punch the clock; as to the future he asked whether I could afford to resign and allow my college classmates to forge ahead of me. When he said that there would not be any change in working conditions, I resigned and, without a job, returned to New York City.

What I have recorded about Parke Davis is not a criticism of that company in particular. Had I joined any of the five or six other leading pharmaceutical manufacturing companies of that day my experience would have been the same. The year 1910 was long before the discovery of vitamins, hormones, or chemotherapeutic agents. Laboratories for control of purity and potency of extracts were essential and all leading firms had them. I would have been equally out of place in any of those laboratories.

Within a month of my return to New York I was told of a possible position in a new laboratory that had been completed and was ready for occupancy. St. Luke's Hospital at Amsterdam Avenue and 114th Street had built a third-floor addition to a building that housed several laboratories occupied by pathologists. Dr. Francis Carter Wood and Dr. Carl Vogel of Columbia University Medical School were looking for a chemist to assist them with chemical questions. There was just one difficulty, money, and Dr. Nellis B. Foster of the same school solved that problem.

Dr. Foster was interested in chemical changes in patients who had diabetes. He came to the laboratory infrequently and performed some determinations on the urine of patients in the hospital. Also he was custodian of a small amount of money that was to be spent for research. From this sum he arranged to give me $30 a month— on a temporary basis.

The pros and cons of this situation were clearly visible. I was to work alone on projects of my own choosing. I was available for consultation to members of the hospital staff and administration but I would not carry out routine analyses in connection with patients. Obviously my future rested solely on my ability to create work of value to the hospital. There was no policy concerning tenure or salary and no discussion of possible other members of the staff. This laboratory was not an addition to a department of chemistry already in existence. It was a new venture without any precedent or plans. The project appeared to be a gamble with heavy odds against a successful career. In spite of the many omissions there was one feature that was most attractive. This was a notebook in which I was asked to list any chemical or apparatus required for the work. What more could one expect or ask for? I accepted the opportunity and on February 1, 1911, began work on isolation of the hormone of the thyroid gland.

The adrenal medulla and the thyroid were the first two endocrine glands to relinquish some of their mysteries to the chemist. The beginning was made during the concluding years of the nineteenth century. In the decade 1890–1900 there were many able men on the faculty of the medical school of the University of Freiburg, Germany. Head of the department of physiological chemistry was the distinguished Professor Eugen Baumann. In 1894, Emminghaus, professor of psychiatry at Freiburg, and Reinholt, his young associate, published a paper that demonstrated a favorable influence of thyroid substance on certain goiters. This work came to the attention of the professor of surgery, Dr. Kraske, who, in turn, requested Baumann to prepare stable preparations of the active material of the thyroid gland for use in clinical medicine.

Preliminary experiments with the thyroid glands of sheep

19

showed that the physiologic activity was not lost when the glands were boiled in acid or heated with alkali. Baumann then found that much of the inert material was broken down and made soluble after boiling with 10 percent sulfuric acid but that a brown residue still carried the original activity of the whole gland. In the spring of 1895, Dr. Roos joined Baumann in an investigation of the thyroid gland. During this work they determined the amount of phosphorus in desiccated thyroid. This analysis required fusion with sodium hydroxide. In the fall of 1895, Baumann fused some material from the thyroid gland with sodium hydroxide and then made the solution acidic with nitric acid. Iodine was liberated. Had he used any acid other than nitric, the presence of iodine in the thyroid gland would have remained entirely unsuspected. Baumann was fully conscious of the importance of the observation, but he did not try to derive prestige as a prophet. Quite without pretension he said, "When I first made this observation I believed anything else rather than that the iodine belonged to my substance." As soon as this determination of iodine had been checked, Baumann analyzed the brown fraction obtained by boiling the thyroid gland with 10 percent sulfuric acid. This material contained 9.30 percent of iodine and 0.56 percent of phosphorus; it was designated iodothyrin.

Publication of Baumann's discovery of iodine in the thyroid gland brought great prestige to the medical school at Freiburg, but in less than a year after his discovery, Baumann died from a heart condition.

For several years, interest in the thyroid gland continued to grow. Although many investigators believed that the iodine-containing compound was associated with the physiologic activity of the gland, this had not been shown, and the significance of Baumann's discovery went unexplained for nineteen years.

The four months that I spent at Parke Davis and Co. afforded one important conclusion that determined the future direction of the investigation. It seemed best to utilize the surprising contribution of Baumann and attempt to isolate the compound that contained iodine. In 1895 nothing was known about the function of iodine in the body. It was known that in patients who did not possess an active thyroid gland edema frequently was a sign of the

condition and it was suggested that the thyroid gland was a detoxi-
fying agent.

The nature of the toxin controlled by the thyroid gland and the
relation of iodine to the gland were matters of surmise but they
increased the need to replace speculation with hard facts concerning the mysterious compound revealed by Baumann.

One other reason that decided the pathway of the project for
me was the presence of iodine in the much-disputed compound.
This was a secure and characteristic label that greatly simplified
the problem, for if the percentage of iodine was determined in any
product separated from the thyroid gland then the amount of
purification would be known.

Since the accurate determination of iodine was a prerequisite
for progress, I had carried out some research to increase the
accuracy of this method while I was in Detroit and this problem
was explored further at St. Luke's Hospital. This work was completed and published in 1912.

The chemical work during the three years in New York can
be described as a steady but slow accumulation of results. To an
optimist the progress was gratifying. The iodine-containing compound in the thyroid gland was clearly shown to be linked to protein; to isolate Baumann's compound in pure form free of all other
components of protein would require some relatively severe treatment. Baumann, as has been mentioned, used boiling 10 percent
sulfuric acid for his preparation of iodothyrin, but I chose repeated
treatment with hot dilute sodium and barium hydroxides, followed
by separation of acid insoluble material. This is described in Chapter
4; at this point I shall record progress of another kind. I refer to
my social status and the development of the instinct for exploration
in myself.

As time passed the hospital found the money to raise my salary
to $1200 a year. This was sufficient for a bachelor, and worry over
material matters came to an end. In the fall of 1912 an event of first
importance changed the course of my life. I acquired a partner who
made the difference between existing and living. In Chapter 2, I
mentioned as a fellow member of Sigma Alpha Epsilon, Walter
Phelps Hall. He came to Columbia as a graduate student in the
department of history. We became close friends, spent vacations

together, took canoe trips, and visited in each other's homes. Walter was the son of a Presbyterian minister in Newburgh, New York. He had graduated from Yale with a Phi Beta Kappa key, and had traveled widely in this country and abroad. He was a man of wide understanding and learning. His greatest interests were in history, sociology, political philosophy, and people. He knew very little about chemistry, physics, or other fields of science. He could not change a tire on an automobile, but he could hold a large audience spellbound with a lecture on Garibaldi, his favorite historical character. He was tolerant of the shortcomings of men and exerted a strong influence for good in the lives of all who came to know him.

Walter enjoyed walking through stores and making purchases. He did not like to cook. My likes and dislikes were the opposite, so shopping for groceries was his job and cooking was mine. In the fall of 1912 we signed a lease for a two-room kitchenette apartment at the Bancroft Apartment House on 123rd Street.

Life was indeed pleasant. After dinner we frequently played dominoes. I kept track of the games won and lost. As the months passed one would be five or six games ahead but soon the other would be in the lead. Many years later I came across the notebook that held the scores. On the flyleaf was this note: "I hereby acknowledge E. C. Kendall to be my domino peer. We are giving up this damn game for chess." It was signed W. P. Hall.

For recreation I frequently attended the opera. Immediately behind the last row of seats on the main floor was a large area for those who remained standing. A polished brass tube almost three inches in cross section was placed, shoulder high, just behind the last row of seats. Those who came early could find some support on this tube. The price of seats in the back row was $6.00. The price for standing room was $1.50. *Madame Butterfly, Tristan und Isolde,* and *Lohengrin* were my favorite operas; Geraldine Farrar was my favorite singer.

St. Luke's Hospital was and is situated in a relatively small community that included the Cathedral of St. John, Columbia University, and an adequate supply of restaurants and stores to answer the everyday needs of the population. My six years of residence at Columbia had made me a member of the neighborhood, and one important reason for my willingness to leave Parke Davis and seek

22

a new career in New York City was that this section of the city was home for me. The inspiring dignity of Low Memorial Library of Columbia University and the reassuring atmosphere created by the massive architecture on the campus, the hospital, and the cathedral, created a sense of security that was not only helpful but essential for one whose position was as tenuous as mine. In some respects I was but one of those who were engaged in the attempt to become well known and "accepted" through their own efforts to create. I refer to young poets, musicians, writers, sculptors, painters, and educators. However, there was this difference. My future rested not on the creation of something beautiful, or in arousing emotional appreciation of the written word or music. The sole basis of my success was the ability to create a procedure by which an unknown substance could be separated in pure crystalline form from a complex of blood, fat, and glandular tissue to which it was firmly attached. Furthermore, the new compound would have to be of importance as a useful agent for the treatment of patients.

In addition, I was but one of a group engaged in exactly the same adventure in other laboratories; who would be the first to succeed? Finally, how long could I expect St. Luke's Hospital to support a young man engaged in an enterprise that involved so many imponderables?

My own reaction to this situation was far from fear and worry. I was not a director of research that was to be carried out by others. No one separated me from direct contact with the actual operations in the laboratory. I alone devised the daily schedule of work and I alone carried out that schedule. The results of the work brought their own daily reward and built a strong confidence in my ability to succeed.

There were of course many days when hope was deferred and serious questions arose concerning work in the laboratory that would have shaken or shattered the confidence of anyone who was less determined. These were the times when it was so important to me to have the moral support of someone who had the sterling character of Walter P. Hall.

By the year 1913 I had devised a method by which Baumann's compound was increased from 1 part in 500 parts of glandular tissue to 1 part in 5 or 6 parts of inert material. This is to say, the

23

concentration was about 100 times. For a criterion of physiological activity I secured a dog in a so-called metabolism cage and determined the amounts of nitrogen excreted daily in the urine and feces when the dog was given a constant intake of food. On a diet that maintained the animal at a nearly constant weight, the excretion of nitrogen was surprisingly constant at a level slightly below the intake of nitrogen in the food. If thyroid gland was added to the diet and all other conditions were kept without change, the excretion of nitrogen increased suddenly during the second day of the experiment. At the same time the pulse rate increased markedly and the character of the pulse changed to a sharp pounding quality.

When it was shown that samples of purified fractions from the thyroid gland produced the same response in the dog and also that these samples could be heated in an autoclave to 110 degrees C. in alkaline solution, I became convinced that the project could be carried to a successful conclusion. To confirm the physiological activity indicated by the results on the dog, I was eager to test this purified fraction on patients.

Through the assistance of Dr. Wood and Dr. Vogel arrangements were made to expand the scope of my project to include treatment of patients. The prospect of applying the fruits of my work in the chemical laboratory to clinical medicine pleased me very much. It was a long step beyond any such possibility at Parke Davis. My position in the chemical investigation of the thyroid gland would be strengthened by enlisting the cooperation of physicians.

A patient in the women's ward, Mrs. M., was suffering from lack of activity of her thyroid gland, and I was permitted to give her whatever products from my work seemed desirable. A record of the treatment was entered on the history of the patient, and daily "hospital rounds" were made. Mrs. M. responded in a highly satisfactory manner. A picture taken after treatment showed that her previous dull, stupid expression had been replaced with a bright and alert look. It seemed that I had widened the basis of my support at St. Luke's.

I was on high ground. Baumann's iodine-containing compound had been separated in concentrated form, and the physiological activity was still present. Further application of the method of purification almost certainly would afford a pure crystalline compound! Or so it seemed to me, but I soon found this conclusion to be naive and untenable. I was now dealing not with glands and chemical reagents but with personalities. The senior attending physicians were pleased with the obvious relief of the signs and symptoms of myxedema, but their reaction was wholly unexpected. Instead of saying, "Splendid, where do we go from here?" their only reaction was "So what?" Among the interns and younger attending physicians there was open and outspoken hostility. I was only a little, if any, older than they were, and they could not accept the fact that any worthwhile clinical result could come out of my work in the laboratory. They were in the hospital to gain experience in the treatment of patients. They wanted to see patients with as many different diseases as possible. They did not want any beds occupied by patients who were involved in clinical research conducted by a young man who did not have an M.D.

This traumatic experience was followed by four incidents that caused a great change in my life.

The first of these was that the administrator of the hospital sent me a letter, and with it a small box of cereal. The tone of the letter was that of a big-time boss giving orders to a lowly henchman. He directed me to analyze the cereal and then asked how the physicians in the hospital could be expected to treat patients unless they knew what they were giving. I threw the letter and the cereal into the wastebasket, but I wondered who had asked the administrator to send the letter. I was certain he had not acted on his own volition.

The second incident occurred because Dr. Rufus Cole, who was chief physician at the hospital of the Rockefeller Institute, became much interested in my work on the thyroid gland. He told me that Rockefeller Institute had reviewed the work of Dr. David Marine on the effect of iodine in relation to the development of goiter and suggested that I should see Dr. Simon Flexner, director of the Institute. Dr. Cole made an appointment for me with Dr. Flexner, and I was in his office at the arranged time. I summarized the work I had done and told of my hopes for the future. Dr. Flexner made no effort to conceal his skepticism of my ability to isolate Baumann's compound. He said, "Young man, it is not easy to get into the Rockefeller Institute. When we want to have someone come with us we will do whatever is necessary to get him, but otherwise it is not possible to join this Institute. Now, what you should do is to go on and separate the iodine-containing compound in pure crystalline form." Obviously he was satisfied that such a feat was completely beyond my power. I did not argue the matter. I stood up and said, "Yes sir, I shall do just that." I did not like what Dr. Flexner said and I disliked the way he said it. However, his remarks only strengthened my determination to isolate Baumann's compound, if it was humanly possible to do so.

The next incident was a conversation with Dr. Wood in which he remarked that on summer trips to Europe in the past he had visited laboratories in various medical schools, where he would meet the members of the laboratory staff and would make an offer for one of them to come to America and work in his laboratory. That seemed to be a fair-enough arrangement, but then he went on to say that after he had "milked" the laboratory assistant he would let him go. I was not working for Dr. Wood but I was in his laboratory and I wondered how long it would be before I, too, was "milked."

The final decisive incident was that in late October 1913 I found a letter on my desk in the laboratory. It was not stamped; it had been delivered by Miss Susan Wood, Dr. Wood's secretary. The gist of it was that my salary for 1914 would be the same as it had been in 1913.

And so ended my efforts to carry out research in biochemistry in an institution that was not interested in research.

Four

The Mayo Clinic and Thyroxin

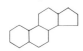

IN THE SUMMER of 1913 I visited friends in Columbia, Missouri. While there I met Professor Clarence M. Jackson of the medical school of the University of Missouri. Professor Jackson was in the process of moving to the medical school of the University of Minnesota. He had just returned from a trip to Minneapolis and planned to move there in the fall of 1913. During our conversation he told me about a new building that was to be occupied in the near future by the Mayo Clinic in Rochester, Minnesota.

He was acquainted with Dr. Louis B. Wilson, director of laboratories at the Mayo Clinic, and suggested I write to him concerning a position. Professor Jackson believed that Dr. Wilson wanted to enlarge research at the Mayo Clinic by addition of a laboratory for biochemistry.

In a letter to Dr. Wilson I described the work I had completed and asked for an interview. Dr. Wilson was interested and an interview was arranged.

On an afternoon in early November, 1913, in Rochester, Minnesota, Dr. Wilson was conducting a group of about fifteen visitors around the "new clinic building." From a modest beginning in 1889, the clinic in recent years had been expanding rapidly. Following the installation of a new X-ray section and new laboratories for clinical pathology, additional space became necessary. As construc-

27

tion progressed, visiting physicians were taken on tours of inspection. Dr. Wilson and Dr. Henry S. Plummer regarded these tours as time well spent, since the new building was the tangible evidence of a departure in medical education, and from the beginning the lists of visitors included many prominent names. The most distinguished member of this particular tour was Dr. Herman Biggs, head of the New York State Department of Health, but among the group was a young man of twenty-seven—myself—who had come to Rochester to discuss a position in the new laboratories. The work was in the field of biochemistry and had to do with the hormone of the thyroid gland.

Dr. Wilson took the members of the party through the rooms on the first three floors. He pointed out that these floors were utilized for the examination and treatment of patients, but that the fourth floor was of interest for other reasons. On the south side of this floor was a large space for the library. The Section of Publications and the office of the librarian were in the front of the building, and the north wing was devoted to laboratories.

As Dr. Wilson came to the end of the corridor he said, "Here we have reserved space for a biochemical laboratory if we decide to expand in this direction. No detailed plans have been prepared. The space will remain unfinished until the plans are drawn by the head of the new department."

Dr. Biggs and the other visitors agreed that this was a wise decision. I said nothing, but my thoughts were projected far into the future.

My visit was not related to plans for a new laboratory, but to whether the Mayo Clinic, which was a new venture in group medicine, would add a deparment devoted to research in biochemistry. Dr. Plummer and Dr. Wilson believed that the time was ripe for the new type of work. They had carried on a joint study concerning the relationship of morphologic changes of the thyroid gland to clinical symptoms. The results of the chemical investigation that I described to them seemed to fit into their work in a convincing manner. Many conferences were held. Members of the staff concerned with the diagnosis and treatment of diseases of the thyroid gland were consulted, and a widespread interest in the field was manifested. Consideration of the question extended over a week, but at the end the highest echelon in the administration decided against expanding the clinic's activities into research in biochemistry.

However, among those especially interested in diseases of the thyroid was Dr. Charles Horace Mayo, who, with his brother, Dr. William James Mayo, directed the Mayo Clinic. When Dr. Plummer and Dr. Wilson explained my work to him, the situation was reversed, and I was asked to come to Rochester as soon as a room on the fourth floor could be prepared. The new research in biochemistry began on February 1, 1914, in a room at the northeast corner, just across the corridor from the unfinished rooms reserved for a future biochemical laboratory.

The clinical and other sections did not move in until the second week of March. For six weeks I climbed over piles of plaster and building debris, the only member of the staff in the new building.

I did not arrive empty-handed. The chemical investigations that I had carried on for almost three and a half years, first at Parke Davis and then at St. Luke's Hospital, had shown that the treatment of thyroid glands with a dilute solution of sodium hydroxide hydrolyzed proteins and gave an aqueous solution of the iodine-containing compounds. The addition of acid caused separation of a relatively small fraction that contained about half of the total iodine. This simple process afforded an effective concentration of the iodine-containing compound. All the physiologic activity was present in this "acid-insoluble" material.

The new laboratory was equipped with apparatus necessary for carrying out two projects. The first was the isolation of the iodine-containing compound believed to the hormone of the thyroid gland. The second was the determination of the acid-insoluble fraction in thyroid glands removed surgically at the Mayo Clinic, and correlation of these data with histologic and clinical studies on patients.

One morning, after the work had progressed for some weeks, a member of the Section of Roentgenology brought into the laboratory a small box that contained gallstones. In X rays he had found that the shadows cast by the stones were not uniform. Some stones gave a dark shadow, others did not. He suggested that a chemical analysis might show why this was so. The problem was discussed, the box was left on the laboratory table, and the man departed.

At the time this seemed a minor incident, but the request for assistance from an important section of the clinic raised fundamental questions. On the one hand, there was the strong inclination to be of service and thus broaden intramural connections. Moreover, here was a chance to hedge, to counterbalance the hazards of research with the certainty that comes from the use of classic methods of analysis. Why not make a contribution that would be of interest to the internist, the surgeon, and the roentgenologist and at the same time would be devoid of any risk or failure?

On the other hand, the work would require time. Who would continue exploration of the chemical nature of the acid-insoluble fraction of the thyroid gland? Should the new "Section of Biochemistry" demonstrate its importance to the clinic through cooperation with one and all who sought its help? Or should I place first things first and limit my efforts to research? If I maintained a relentless pursuit of a fixed objective—isolation of the hormone of the thyroid gland—anything that delayed the work was to be avoided. What was the best answer?

My first reaction was to leave the box of gallstones on the table and to proceed with the work that had been interrupted by the visitor. This in itself was an answer, for the longer the box remained on the table the less were the chances it would be opened.

A short time later this incident was brought to a close in a clear and decisive manner. Dr. Wilson frequently visited the laboratory and asked how the work was progressing. One day he saw the little box and wanted to know what was inside. I told him about the request of the roentgenologist and his feeling that the work was very important.

Dr. Wilson said, "Son, you were brought here to do research of the first quality. The analysis of gallstones is not important, and I do not want you to do it. I shall return this box to its owner and shall expect you to carry on with investigation of the hormone of the thyroid gland."

The consequences of this event determined my future for the next thirty-seven years.

All research work has its ups and downs, but the spring, summer, and fall of 1914 were a steady procession of ups. By June the laboratory was well organized and efficient, with Miss Helen Pharo as its first technician. Determinations of iodine, further hydrolysis of the acid-insoluble fraction, and separation of material with an iodine content of 10, then 20, and finally 30 percent held almost certain promise that the objective would be reached.

While Dr. Wilson and Dr. Plummer were in contact with the laboratory and knew in general what was being accomplished, other members of the clinic did not, and by October it had become evident, by way of the grapevine, that this state of affairs was causing questions. The solution seemed to be the presentation of a statement about the work at a meeting of the staff, and this was well received.

November and December of 1914 brought the climax of the investigation. The amount of iodine in the acid-insoluble fraction steadily increased until it reached 47 percent. This suggested that at least some of the material might be separated in crystalline form by the use of a suitable solvent. Ethanol was tried. On the evening of December 23, 1914, the sample of acid-insoluble fraction with the highest percentage of iodine was dissolved in a small amount of alcohol. The sample was so readily soluble that it seemed desirable to concentrate the solution to a small volume. I placed the beaker on a steam bath and sat down to wait until most of the alcohol had evaporated. While I was waiting, I fell asleep. The time that elapsed could not have been long, but when I awoke all the alcohol had evaporated. On the bottom of the small glass container was a white crust and around this a ring of yellowish, waxy material. If crystallization from alcohol was to be achieved, it would be necessary to start over. Alcohol was added. The waxy material dissolved, but the white crust remained insoluble, even in hot alcohol. Some unforeseen separation had been accomplished. There were two possibilities: either the white crust contained more iodine than the original material or it contained less. In the first case, the new white product would be a substantial advance. The crust could be a single substance; it could be an almost pure compound. In the second case, removal of the white crust would result in enrichment of the iodine content of the waxy material.

Which possibility was correct could be found by analyzing the

31

white crust for iodine, but the hour was late and separation of the acid-insoluble material into two distinctly different fractions appeared to be progress sufficient for one day.

Analysis of the white crust the next morning provided a definite answer. The material contained 60 percent iodine. It was the first almost pure preparation of the hormone of the thyroid gland. The process by which it had been obtained was so simple and the climax had come so gradually that it was difficult to realize that this was the end of the project. It had required four years and four months. During the rest of the day, December 24, more of the acid-insoluble fraction was prepared for crystallization from ethanol, and the solubilities of the new compound in various solvents were tested. The iodine compound retained the properties of the acid-insoluble fraction. It was soluble in water in the presence of sodium hydroxide; it was precipitated by the addition of acid.

On Christmas morning, some of the white crust was dissolved in ethanol that contained a small amount of sodium hydroxide. Addition of a few drops of acetic acid precipitated the material in fine crystalline form. It was a single substance with a high melting point.

Throughout the investigation physiologic activity was determined on samples of the acid-insoluble material and the activity was found to be proportional to the percentage of iodine. It was quite certain, therefore, that the crystalline iodine-containing compound also would possess physiologic activity. Sufficient crystalline material was used to show that this was true. This brought to a close the first stage of the investigation.

The year 1914 had been one of unqualified success. Insofar as separation of more of the iodine-containing compound was concerned, the year 1915 was a complete failure. It was, however, a time of growth for the Section of Biochemistry. In the spring, detailed plans were prepared for the utilization of the unfinished rooms across the corridor. They were to be devoted to preparation of the hormone of the thyroid gland on a large scale.

Throughout 1914 the starting material had been desiccated thyroid gland. This had been treated with sodium hydroxide in Pyrex glass flasks, and the acid-insoluble fraction had been hydrolyzed with barium hydroxide in large nickel crucibles. This procedure limited the amount that could be treated, and it was decided to remove this bottleneck by using large metal tanks for the initial hydrolysis. This entailed much research, since the new equipment appeared to destroy the hormone. Eventually it was shown that iron and copper did destroy physiologic activity, but porcelain or nickel did not. Fifteen months from the time the first crystals were obtained, most of the difficulties had been removed and a satisfactory method devised by which a steady supply of the hormone was prepared.

The Section of Biochemistry was accepted as an important part of the clinic. The chemical investigation of surgical specimens of thyroid glands furnished interesting information that correlated well with the studies of Drs. Wilson and Plummer.

Treatment of patients with the hormone of the thyroid gland in crystalline form produced astonishing results. Two outstanding cases concerned a girl ten years old and a woman in her fifties. The girl was thirty-seven inches in height and weighed thirty-seven pounds. Both somatic and mental growth were retarded. Her picture was taken, showing her infantile-looking face, while she was holding her doll. She received therapy with the thyroid hormone and was sent home for six months. When she returned it was difficult to believe that she was the same child. She had grown four inches and had changed mentally into a bright, responsive person. At the end of a year she returned again. She had grown two more inches, and when her picture was taken in the dress she wore originally, the long sleeves came only to the elbow, and the hem was above her knees.

The woman had been sent to the clinic by a judge in Illinois. She was accompanied by her sister and a nurse. She had been diagnosed as mentally incompetent. If this finding was confirmed by the clinic and a hopeless prognosis given, the judge would assign her to an institution and divide her estate among her relatives. The patient was found to be suffering from myxedema. Her skin was dry and scaly, her face was puffy, and she had a vacant, stupid expression. Administration of the thyroid hormone abated the edema, brought back her usual keenness of mind, and restored her to her former activities.

These patients were presented at a meeting of the staff. They were dramatic and convincing evidence that biochemistry could be of practical use in clinical medicine.

These and many similar results of the use of the hormone with patients raised the question of the physiologic action of the new compound. What physiologic processes were affected and what chemical reactions were modified? Was the iodine-containing compound the only active substance in the thyroid gland? How much of the compound circulated in the bloodstream of the human being? How much was made by the thyroid gland in a day? What was the chemical structure of the compound? Could it be prepared synthetically? These were some of the most obvious questions. A new chapter in medicine had been opened. The future of the Section of Biochemistry was full of promise.

Progress in the work resulted in my appointment to the staff of the Mayo Clinic and an income that allowed me to think of marriage. December 30, 1915, was the date of my wedding with Rebecca Kennedy of Buffalo, New York, and on the same day in 1965 we happily celebrated our golden anniversary.

In 1916 I was asked to present a paper at the plenary session of the annual meeting of the Federation of American Societies for Experimental Biology in New York City. It was a satisfaction to comply. The title of the paper was "Isolation in Crystalline Form of the Iodine-Containing Compound of the Thyroid Gland." The chairman of the meeting was Dr. Simon Flexner.

When the method of separation of the hormone had been devised, it became possible to carry out experiments on animals. These were continued for many years and entailed a great expansion of the work in the section. Proteins were hydrolyzed to yield amino acids that were injected intravenously into animals, together with an excess of the thyroid hormone. The urine and blood were analyzed for amino acids, urea, and ammonia, but no direct influence of the hormone could be shown.

Among the first questions to be investigated were the composition and structure of the hormone. In 1916 micromethods for the analysis of organic compounds were not generally available, and since almost two-thirds of the weight of the hormone was iodine, large samples were required for the determination of carbon, hydrogen, and nitrogen. Help was now needed to carry on the investigation in the field of organic chemistry, and Arnold E. Osterberg, a recent graduate of the University of Washington, joined the section.

The hormone was analyzed and was found to have the following composition, expressed in percentages: carbon, hydrogen, oxygen, nitrogen and iodine, respectively 22.37, 1.65, 8.73, 2.23, and 65.02. Analysis of the sulfate salt indicated a molecular weight of 565. This value and the percentage composition permitted determination of the empirical formula as $C_{11}H_{14}O_3NI_3$. When the hormone was heated with sodium hydroxide the volatile compound indole was formed; this suggested that indole was the organic nucleus to which the iodine was attached. The structural formula tentatively assigned was tri-iodohexahydro-oxindolepropionic acid.

This structure was first suggested in 1918. The chemical formula was obviously too cumbersome to be used as the name of the hormone, and much thought was given to the derivation of a suitable short designation. While this was under discussion, Osterberg and I, en route to a meeting of the American Chemical Society, were walking up and down the platform in the LaSalle Street railroad station in Chicago. I remarked that "thyroxindole" would be descriptive but was too long.

Osterberg suggested, "Why not drop the last syllable and call it thyroxin?"

A definitive paper describing the isolation of thyroxin and giving the details of its chemical structure and properties was published in 1918, but even before its publication the next step—synthesis of the hormone—had been started. To produce a compound that possessed the structure assigned to thyroxin required preparation of a series of compounds hitherto unknown. After several years of work and some initial failures a compound was made synthetically that was identical with the nucleus that had been assigned tentatively to the nucleus of thyroxin. The achievement of this objective brought both the satisfaction that comes with success and the promise that thyroxin would be prepared synthetically.

The only remaining problem, so it seemed, was to attach the three atoms of iodine to the nucleus. One atom could be added without difficulty; after much further work, two atoms were attached; but the addition of a third atom was not achieved. The difficulties encountered did not stop the work, although successive failures would probably have accumulated to such a formidable extent as to necessitate a thorough survey and check of all the results. Unfortunately,

35

the day-to-day progress was sufficient to allay any suspicion that all was not well: ultimate success, although delayed, seemed assured.

In the spring of 1926, work on the synthesis of thyroxin in the Section of Biochemistry at the Mayo Foundation was suddenly stopped and then entirely abandoned. Up to that time obstacles that appeared to be complete barriers had been overcome, but now a situation arose to which there was no answer. The objective had been reached in another laboratory.

The first warning came from Dr. H. D. Dakin, one of the editors of the *Journal of Biological Chemistry*. I had submitted a manuscript describing some chemical properties of the compound that we believed was the nucleus of thyroxin. The manuscript was accepted, but Dr. Dakin wrote a letter to me in which he suggested that publication be delayed because of some new work that he had done. He had made the observation that indole was not the nucleus of thyroxin but rather that indole was formed during the treatment of the hormone with sodium hydroxide. He also had isolated tyrosine by severe hydrolysis of thyroxin. Finally, Dr. Dakin's letter stated that Dr. C. R. Harington, of University College, London, had separated and identified the nucleus of thyroxin. Harington's results were published without delay, and since they established the structure of thyroxin in an unequivocal manner, additional work on iodo derivatives of indole was abandoned.

The readjustment required to meet this situation was a severe test for me as well as for the staff members. One response was typical of the loyal support extended by the clinic. It was the custom to hold dinner meetings of all staff members at intervals, and at such a meeting I requested the opportunity to describe the new situation. I reviewed the work on the synthesis of thyroxin and explained the failure to identify the thyroxin nucleus. This had resulted from the loss of traces of iodine during analysis of the hormone. Determination of known amounts of iodide added to organic matter gave results that were 100 percent accurate, but when thyroxin was fused with sodium hydroxide very small amounts of iodoindole were lost by volatilization. This fact was unknown throughout the investigation, but I was able to demonstrate it after Harington's work was published. The percentages of carbon, hydrogen, oxygen, nitrogen, and iodine in triiodohexahydro-oxindole propionic acid (thyroxin) are almost the same as those in the tetra-iodo derivative of thyronine, the name given by Harington to the nucleus of the hormone. The close approximation of the content of iodine in the tri-iodo compound (65.02 percent) to that in the tetra-iodo substance was coincidental, but it effectively obscured the structure of thyroxin.

During my talk to the staff I pointed out that the isolation of thyroxin was a success that belonged to all members of the staff and failure to complete the synthesis a loss of prestige that must be shared by all; I also expressed my regret and concern that time had brought about such a situation. At the end of the talk Dr. Wilson asked Dr. Plummer whether he wished to make any remarks. Dr. Plummer's response was perhaps as important for my future at the clinic as was the incident with the gallstones. He arose in a deliberate manner and said, "The height of the tower in the new clinic building is two hundred and twenty-seven feet above the sidewalk." The meeting adjourned.

The failure to synthesize thyroxin was a bitter disappointment, but other phases of the investigation helped to restore confidence and renew initiative. A method for the determination of iodine in blood was devised, and the first published work on this subject came from the Mayo Clinic. A seasonal variation in the iodine content of the thyroid gland had been shown by Frederick Fenger. This knowledge was extended at the clinic to the seasonal variations of the acid-insoluble fraction and of thyroxin.

Dr. W. M. Boothby and his associates at the clinic made many important studies on the clinical use of thyroxin. Patients with myxedema were chosen to show the influence of thyroxin on the basal metabolic rate and to determine the rate at which the body lost the effect of thyroxin after its administration was ceased. Still other investigations dealt with changes in protein metabolism induced by thyroxin.

It seemed desirable to gather together all the results that had been published concerning thyroxin, and the opportunity was provided when the American Chemical Society asked me to prepare a monograph on the subject. *Thyroxine,* published in 1928, was No. 47 of the American Chemical Society Series; it is also the source of the information on thyroxin in this chapter. The spelling "thyroxine" was Harington's suggestion; today both spellings are accepted.

Five

New Work in Biochemistry

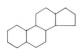

THE 1920s WERE marked by rapid expansion at the Mayo Clinic. The investigations concerned with the thyroid gland were widespread and the contributions from research were fundamental. Dr. Plummer's use of iodides for the treatment of hyperthyroidism reduced the surgical mortality rates to a percentage hitherto impossible to achieve. The Mayo Clinic, long recognized for excellence as a surgical clinic, assumed a position of first rank among medical centers throughout the world. The laboratory division of the clinic was organized with a Laboratory Society that was given equal status with the Surgical Society and the Clinical Society.

A local chapter of the professional scientific fraternity Sigma Xi was installed, and in 1928 the clinic was asked to form a chapter of the Society for Experimental Biology and Medicine, to which more than a dozen members of the staff already belonged. After thorough discussion, however, the staff decided instead to organize a research club that would serve the needs of the clinic but would not be affiliated with any national society.

The Research Club, of which I was the chairman for its first twenty-three years, did not have a charter, bylaws, or dues. Meetings were held once a month from October to May inclusive. The program always consisted of three papers, on subjects related to research that

39

had been carried out at the Mayo Foundation. Each paper occupied twenty minutes, with ten minutes allowed for discussion.

The club had several valuable functions. It brought together in a social way laboratory workers who did not meet on any other occasion. It gave laboratory technicians an opportunity to hear presentations of results that they had helped obtain, thus contributing to morale. It was a splendid forum for the presentation and defense of work soon to be published. Statements made before the club were frequently modified before publication. The meetings gave young researchers an opportunity to learn to present and summarize a scientific paper and to prepare lantern slides. The high level attained served to eliminate papers that were inferior, and many fundamental contributions in physiology, bacteriology, biophysics, and biochemistry were presented.

It was my good fortune to become a member of the staff of the Mayo Clinic very early—even before the establishment of the Mayo Foundation. At that time the entire staff was a group with common interests. Dr. Will (Dr. W. J. Mayo) and Dr. Charlie (Dr. C. H. Mayo) were in their full strength as men and surgeons, and the example that they set was without blemish. Their lives were devoted to each other, to their families, and to medicine. Medicine to them meant the Mayo Clinic, and they were most generous in efforts to establish a strong loyalty among members of the staff.

Dr. Charlie was always interested in the chemical work on the thyroid gland. He alone had been its sponsor and he strongly supported the development of the research. He was an effective public relations man and often referred to thyroxin in papers and addresses.

All members of the staff were conscious that it was Dr. Will who ran the Mayo Clinic. Anything that brought it prestige was of immediate concern to him. Prior to the work on thyroxin he had not been interested in chemistry. When he saw the clinical changes wrought with thyroxin and realized what it meant to have this contribution come from the clinic, he became a staunch patron and gave full support to research in biochemistry.

In my scrapbook are many notes from Dr. Will, written to express his appreciation of work that came from the laboratory. They were sent to a young man just starting out in an attempt to show that research in biochemistry was worth while. Coming from a man who had made an outstanding success of his life, they were morale builders of the first order.

One consequence of the publication of the work on thyroxin was to draw attention to the opportunity for graduate work in biochemistry at the Mayo Foundation. In 1921 I was appointed professor of physiologic chemistry in the Mayo Foundation in the Graduate School of the University of Minnesota. In 1922 Bernard F. McKenzie joined the Section of Biochemistry as a laboratory assistant and during the following thirty years his patience, persistence, and ability were largely responsible for the contributions made by the laboratory.

The influence of thyroxin on the basal metabolic rate was an indication that in some manner thyroxin modified the oxidation of some metabolite or component of the cells in all tissues of the body. The explanation of the influence of thyroxin in terms of chemistry was one of the first objectives of the investigation. In the early 1920s, Dr. William Mansfield Clark, who was recognized as "the father of hydrogen ions," developed methods for the determination of oxidation-reduction potentials. A conference with Dr. Clark convinced me that this lead should be followed up, and as a result investigations in the field of physical chemistry were begun in my laboratory and continued for several years. It seemed possible that a study of the oxidation of cysteine and glutathione would help explain the influence of thyroxin on oxidation in the body.

Cysteine could be purchased, but for our purpose it was necessary to purify it. We decided to prepare cystine from protein. Hair from Dibble's barber shop, at twenty-five cents for a large bag, was the source. McKenzie separated cystine and soon we had a large sample of pure cysteine for use in a study of the oxidation of this important amino acid.

Glutathione could not be purchased. This compound had been isolated, analyzed, and named by Professor F. Gowland Hopkins of Cambridge University in 1921. He had shown that glutamic acid and cysteine are present in the compound, and he believed that the newly separated component of tissue was a dipeptide of these two amino acids. Hence the name "gluta-thione." Glutathione had never been crystallized and attempts to prepare the dipeptide by synthesis had not afforded a crystalline product. The preparation of glutathione in other laboratories had yielded only amorphous material. It was seven years after the isolation of the compound when I decided to prepare glutathione and compare its redox potentials with those of cysteine.

The method devised by Hopkins was followed, except for one modification which eventually was shown to be most important. When yeast is suspended in water, glutathione is retained, attached to the cells. McKenzie and I found that if benzene is present the glutathione is detached and passes almost completely into the aqueous phase. Furthermore, since this occurs at room temperature, the peptide is not destroyed and the amount of extraneous material is reduced to a minimum.

A Sharples centrifuge was installed; glutathione was detached from large quantities of yeast; the cells were removed; and many batches of glutathione were prepared. Minor changes in the method of isolation were made; the time required was shortened and the quality of the product much improved. In the spring of 1929 a concentrated solution of glutathione was placed in a desiccator. After some time it was noted that the appearance of the solution had changed. It was opaque and filled with a white material. Glutathione had separated in crystalline form. A sample of highly purified glutathione was analyzed. The percentage of sulfur was too low, and the percentage of nitrogen too high, for the dipeptide glutamyl cysteine. The analysis was correct for a tripeptide of glutamic acid cysteine and glycine.

The isolation of glutathione in crystalline form and its chemical identification as a tripeptide came as a surprise. Many questions could now be answered, but first it was necessary to finish the chemical identification of the compound. Dr. Harold L. Mason, who had joined the Section of Biochemistry during the preceding months and who had been engaged with problems concerned with determination of glutathione in the blood, now joined McKenzie and me in the work involved in the proof of structure of the tripeptide. Time was important. The International Congress of Physiologists was to meet in Boston, Massachusetts, in August 1929. The meeting would provide an excellent opportunity for presentation of the results, but only a short time remained for submission of papers to be presented. The abstract was sent in time and the paper was well received. Its presentation, however, produced still another surprise.

Professor Hopkins did not attend the Congress, but in the discussion one of his friends reported that during the preceding months Hopkins had separated glutathione in crystalline form and also had found that glutathione is a tripeptide with the structure which we had reported. Professor Hopkins, alerted by his friend, promply dispatched a statement about his results to *Nature*. However, the abstract of our paper in the program of the congress was the first publication of the chemical structure of crystalline glutathione.

Hopkins had shown that in glutathione the carboxyl group of glutamic acid is combined with the amino group of cysteine. Within a short time after the meeting of the congress, Mason, McKenzie, and I published the first of a series of papers* giving the chemical evidence that in glutathione the carboxyl group of the cysteine is attached to the amino group of glycine. The compound therefore is glutamyl-cysteinyl-glycine.

Final proof for the correctness of this structure was furnished by Dr. Harington, discoverer of the thyroxin nucleus, who synthesized glutathione. Still later an elegant method for its preparation was devised by Vincent du Vigneaud, professor of biochemistry at Cornell University Medical School. For reasons that will be evident, no attempt to synthesize glutathione was made at the Mayo Clinic.

* *Journal of Biological Chemistry*, 84:657–675; 87:55–79; 88:409–423.

Six

Beginnings of Adrenal Research

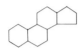

IN THE SPRING of 1929 a letter was received from England that influenced the program of research for the next twenty years. The Hungarian chemist Dr. Albert Szent-Györgyi had isolated small amounts of a compound that was widely distributed in fruits, vegetables, and animals. He had determined the chemical properties of the compound and had suggested the name "hexuronic acid."

The highest concentration of hexuronic acid that Szent-Györgyi had found was in the adrenal cortex, and this gland had been the source for isolation of the new compound. The investigation had proceeded to the point where it was essential to separate sufficient hexuronic acid to permit determination of the chemical structure and physiologic effects of the compound. For this, Szent-Györgyi had made several attempts to secure fresh adrenal glands from packing houses in England, either by prompt delivery of a sufficiently large amount of fresh glands, or by a supply of glands that had been kept in dry ice from the moment they were removed from cattle. Neither of these possibilities was realized. He arranged to have glands collected in Denmark and shipped to Cambridge by air. When these were received he found that the elusive new compound had disappeared. Szent-Györgyi planned to attend the International Congress of Physiology in Boston in August 1929, and some months before that time he wrote me to ask whether it would be possible to

45

join the staff of the biochemical laboratory of the Mayo Foundation as a visiting scientist and to reside in Rochester long enough to complete work on the isolation of hexuronic acid. It was his hope that adrenal glands could be secured from some of the large packing houses in St. Paul, Minnesota.

This matter was referred by Dr. Wilson, who was then director of the Mayo Foundation, to the Board of Governors. They extended an invitation to Szent-Györgyi and his wife to come to Rochester in the fall of 1929. They arrived in September and remained for eight months.

A room on the top floor of the Zumbro Annex was assigned for the work, and the new member of the laboratory was given an assistant, Miss Irma Bair. Regular shipments of fresh bovine adrenal glands were received, and before his departure Szent-Györgyi had isolated several grams of hexuronic acid.

When he left in May 1930 he remarked that he had decided not to investigate further the physiologic properties of hexuronic acid. He had already supplied some of the compound for an investigation of its possible relationship to vitamin C. The report was negative, and since he had made the compound available for chemical and physiologic investigation he was not interested in additional research on hexuronic acid. Furthermore, he said that if I was inclined to work with the new compound he would be happy to have the problem studied in my laboratory.

Szent-Györgyi had sent a sample of hexuronic acid to Professor Walter Haworth of Birmingham University, who had expressed a willingness to investigate the chemical structure of the compound. For some unknown reason this investigation was postponed for nearly two years, and during that period hexuronic acid and vitamin C were shown to be one and the same compound. Then there was a furious attempt in several laboratories to establish the structure of vitamin C.

Some idea of the competition is given by an incident told to me later by Szent-Györgyi. A man from a laboratory in Switzerland went to Szeged, Hungary, where Szent-Györgyi's laboratory was then located, to learn how to separate vitamin C from Hungarian peppers, which had been found to be the best source. The visitor left Szeged by train on a Friday night, taking with him a sample of vitamin C. Immediately on his arrival in the laboratory in Switzerland a series of experiments was carried out. The following Tuesday Szent-Györgyi received by mail a galley proof of a paper that came from the pen of the recent visitor. It contained the evidence for the chemical structure of the vitamin.

Szent-Györgyi's career after his return to Hungary in the summer of 1930 was meteoric. He was made professor of medical chemistry at the University of Szeged and was provided with a new, well-equipped laboratory. Soon after this he built up a group of able scientists and carried out a project concerned with oxidation in the animal organism. Among his assistants was Joseph L. Svirbely, an American of Hungarian parentage, who went to Szeged on a fellowship given by Hungarians who lived in the vicinity of Pittsburgh, Pennsylvania.

Svirbely had just been graduated with the degree of doctor of philosophy from the University of Pittsburgh, where he had worked under Professor C. G. King on the isolation of vitamin C from citrus fruits. Investigation of vitamin C had been carried out in Professor King's laboratory for some years. When Svirbely left Pittsburgh the work on vitamin C was far advanced and the end was within sight.

With Svirbely's arrival in Szeged, Szent-Györgyi changed his mind about further investigation of hexuronic acid. Svirbely was well prepared to investigate the possible relationship between hexuronic acid and vitamin C, since he was familiar with the use of guinea pigs as test animals. Guinea pigs were given 1 milligram of hexuronic acid per day and deprived of vitamin C in their diet. They passed the first week without change. They survived the second week without symptoms; the third week was known to be the crucial one, but this, too, was taken in stride. Hexuronic acid maintained guinea pigs on a scorbutic diet indefinitely. It was vitamin C!

At this same time King and his associates completed the investigations at the University of Pittsburgh. Vitamin C was separated in crystalline form and found to be identical with hexuronic acid.

In his new laboratory in Szeged, Szent-Györgyi continued his investigation on the influence of dicarboxyllic acids on oxidation. In 1937 his contributions were recognized by the Nobel Prize in Physiology and Medicine.

A short time after Szent-Györgyi left Rochester I did carry out further work on the isolation of hexuronic acid from adrenal glands and from cabbages. About 10 grams of the compound was obtained. This was kept in the laboratory for two years. At any time during this interval it would have been available for investigation concerning its antiscorbutic properties. In the end a large part of my sample of hexuronic acid was administered to a patient to see whether it would be excreted unchanged in the urine. It was.

The visit of Szent-Györgyi to Rochester was not confined to the laboratory. He and his wife were socially inclined and enjoyed a wide circle of friends. Among the things bequeathed by Szent-Györgyi to Rochester was a revival of interest in chess. He had seen a chessboard in England arranged for four-handed chess, and from his description such a chessboard was made. While he was in our midst and for many years afterward four-handed chess was played at least once a week, sometimes more often.

The year 1930 was a time of decision; an era had come to a close. During the preceding sixteen years laboratory work in biochemistry had grown from one man in one room to a group of twelve assisted by twenty-three technicians, occupying an entire floor. The projects under investigation extended into many facets of the general field of biochemisry. Biochemistry itself had been enlarged beyond the vision of any of the pioneers at the turn of the century.

As the clinical aspects of the investigation of the thyroid gland were completed, the future program for the Section of Biochemistry came under consideration. Of the projects that had been carried on only investigation of the thyroid gland was of interest to internists or surgeons. In 1930 when other sections and departments in the clinic were being called upon to retrench, was it wise to devote any part of the facilities of the laboratory to work that was not closely related to clinical medicine? Obviously not. However, no time was lost. One of the most important problems in the field of clinical medicine had been opened up while Szent-Györgyi was with us. In January 1930, two papers* in *Science* described the first successful attempt to demonstrate the presence of a hormone of the adrenal cortex. One came from Wilbur W. Swingle's laboratory in Princeton, New Jersey, and the other from Frank Hartman's laboratory at the University of Buf-

---

* W. W. Swingle and J. J. Pfiffner, *Science* 72:76 (1930); F. A. Hartman and Katherine A. Brownell, *Science* 72:75-76 (1930).

falo, New York. Szent-Györgyi and I discussed this work, and I began to form tentative plans for a chemical investigation of the adrenal cortex. Actually, we were already at work in this field. Hundreds of pounds of adrenal glands had been treated for the extraction of hexuronic acid. A wooden press, a large meat grinder, and forty-gallon crocks, which had been used for Szent-Györgyi's work, were now available for other use.

A serious study of the hormones of the adrenal cortex seemed a logical step to follow the investigation of the active agent of the thyroid gland, and no stimulation was needed to place this project on the program with top priority. Stimulation nevertheless was forthcoming. For many years Dr. Leonard G. Rowntree and his associates at the Mayo Clinic had carried on a clinical investigation of Addison's disease. The mortality rate of this disease was close to 100 percent and no treatment, even palliative, was known. Rowntree was most interested in Swingle's extract of the adrenal cortex. He wanted to secure the material and treat those patients who still survived at St. Mary's Hospital. Dr. Swingle's associate, Dr. Pfiffner, came to Rochester for a conference with Dr. Rowntree. Some extract was secured, but the preparation of the hormone was on a small laboratory scale, and only limited amounts were available. Dr. Rowntree appealed to me for preparation of the extract.

It was not difficult to decide what to do, but first the work in the field of physical chemistry was brought to a point at which the results could be published. The investigation of the redox potentials of cysteine, cystine, glutathione, and oxindolepropionic acid was concluded. Some aspects of the work remained obscure, but the results would be of theoretical importance only.

The prospect of work on the adrenal cortex was in strong contrast. Successful treatment of a disease accompanied by a mortality rate of 100 percent was a challenge to a chemical investigation of the adrenal gland. But to me the scope of the project, even in 1930, appeared to be far greater than a treatment of Addison's disease. If the hormone of the adrenal cortex could be isolated and prepared for use in clinical medicine, it should have wide application. Before recording the work on the adrenal cortex, it seems desirable to discuss the nature of this type of study.

Certain aspects of such investigations never are mentioned in scientific publications, and few authors have pointed out either the rich reward or the admission fee associated with this kind of research. From the very start the project is directed toward a "fixed objective." The justification for the expenditure of time and money is to be found solely in attainment of that goal. Some examples are Baeyer's synthesis of indigo; Fisher's synthesis of porphyrins; duVigneaud's isolation and synthesis of the hormones of the post-pituitary gland, oxytocin and vasopresin; Woodward's total synthesis of the steroid nucleus, cholesterol, and cortisone, as well as strychnine and reserpine; and R. R. Williams' separation, identification, and synthesis of thiamine. All these outstanding contributions involved a "fixed objective." They were not incidental to other work or sustained by a program of teaching, writing, or research more significant than the goal itself. They were of primary importance and they held a top priority.

A question seldom asked about such work is: What is the driving force that continues to exert pressure during the five, ten, fifteen, or even twenty years that have been required for the completion of some of these projects?

The answer is not simple and surely is not identical for all research problems. Moreover, it cannot be stated in terms that will be understood by all who chance to read it. Some highly intelligent people cannot see why anyone should want to climb mountains; others cannot comprehend the devotion that has overcome great obstacles to interpret the secrets buried in the ruins of ancient civilizations. Similarly, some businessmen or some classical scholars may not be interested in the advancement of science.

But two components of the drive can be understood and are appreciated by almost everyone. These are a love of whatever things are true and a desire to create something. The scientist hopes to discover a small addition to the accumulated truth of the ages and to create procedures that make this revelation available to all. These hopes constitute a powerful drive that is an inexhaustible source of strength.

The conquest of nature by man can be on the highest plane of endeavor, and the reward of achievement is unique. It cannot be purchased with currency, but to the scientist it is his most cherished possession: it is the memory of the moment when he reached the fixed objective.

What is the admission fee charged those who join the body of scientists who devote their lives to research? This in no sense is restrictive. It is, first, the recognition of the concrete problem; second, the acceptance of the fixed objective as a responsibility; and third, the willingness to devote all possible energy to its attainment without regard to time or expenditure of effort.

In 1930 the problem concerning the adrenal cortex was well defined. It had been amply demonstrated that, although the adrenal medulla is not essential for survival, the cortex of the gland makes at least one hormone without which neither animals nor human beings can be maintained in normal condition. Isolation and chemical identification of the hormone were adopted as the immediate program.

Hormones are well-defined compounds, but until their chemical and physical properties are determined they can be recognized only by their physiologic activity. Problems concerning the function of the adrenal gland and the best method for assay of its extracts could be investigated only by the use of animals. In 1930 all work at the Mayo Clinic that involved animals was carried out at the Institute of Experimental Medicine. There were several advantages and one disadvantage associated with segregation of experimental work on animals. The animals and excellent housing for them were provided; the diet was furnished by the institute, and most important, the surgical operations were performed by Dr. Frank C. Mann. I shall always remain indebted to Dr. Mann for his essential contribution. A large number of dogs had their adrenal glands removed; others their thyroid glands; and a few both the pancreas and the adrenal glands. These animals formed the basis for the investigation concerned with the function of the adrenal cortex and methods for assay of the hormones of that structure. The one disadvantage was the distance (four miles) between the chemical laboratory and the Institute of Experimental Medicine. It was necessary to care for the animals and to give them daily injections of the hormones. For a time this was done by Fellows who made the results of this work the basis of their theses for a graduate degree. On some holidays, such as Christmas, when the men wanted a day or two off, I would take over, feed the dogs, give the injections, and make notes so that the program would not be interrupted. During the first three years, before the procedures were standardized, I took full responsibility for the physiologic work.

At that stage of the investigation, survival of a dog whose adrenal gland had been removed rarely exceeded forty-eight hours unless the animal received adequate treatment. As the adrenalectomized dog approached a critical condition, the time passed slowly, sometimes into the small hours before dawn. At the end of this phase of the investigation I could truthfully say that some portion of every hour of the day and night had been spent at the Institute of Experimental Medicine. The frustration associated with failure to save the dog and the satisfaction that came with successful treatment made a lasting impression on me.

After 1933 the preparation of potent extracts removed the doubts and hazards of work on animals. My presence at the institute was no longer required, for two reasons. The standardization of extracts from the adrenal cortex had become a routine process, and assistants especially trained for this work were available. My days were now spent in the chemical laboratory, but throughout the many years that followed, the experiences associated with the work on animals sustained my conviction that investigation of the adrenal cortex was worth while.

Approach to the chemical investigation of the adrenal cortex was of necessity empirical, and for almost three years little progress was made. Methods for separation of active extracts had been available in the literature since 1929, but this information revealed little more than that the hormone is soluble both in water and in organic solvents, such as ether, chloroform, and benzene. Whether the hormone was present in the fat and lipid fraction or in the aqueous phase had not been disclosed.

We observed that if a dilute aqueous or alcoholic solution of sulfuric acid was added to finely ground adrenal glands and they were pressed to separate the meaty phase, the sulfate would be absorbed by the solid material and the solution would be almost completely free of sulfate.

The aqueous phase was found to be decidedly acid. We were prompted to determine the nature of this organic acid and found that it had the properties of lactic acid. The concentration indicated that there is more of this compound in the adrenal gland than in any equal weight of tissue in the body. This new bit of information suggested a possible relationship of lactic acid to epinephrine. Removal of the adrenal medulla does not cause death, but it seemed possible that the adrenal cortex added something to epinephrine that was essential for life. Extraction of fresh adrenal glands with organic solvents, such as chloroform, resulted in a distribution of epinephrine between the aqueous and organic phases. Determination of epinephrine and lactic acid in the chloroform indicated a 1:1 relationship of these two compounds. Did this mean that one molecule of lactic acid was combined with one molecule of epinephrine? Was it possible that the hormone of the adrenal cortex was a derivative of the hormone of the adrenal medulla? Epinephrine lactate, the salt of the acid and base, would not be soluble in chloroform or benzene, but an ester would be soluble. This derivative, lactyl epinephrine, could be made synthetically, and its physiologic activity could be determined.

Lactyl epinephrine was synthesized in the laboratory and given to a series of adrenalectomized dogs. These animals required close attention. Encouraging results were obtained in some cases, but after several days that terminated at 1:00 or 2:00 A.M., and others that started at 4:00 or 5:00 A.M., it became evident that the hormone of the adrenal cortex is not lactyl epinephrine.

Subsequently, it was shown that, in the presence of lecithin, epinephrine is soluble in chloroform. This fact explained the distribution of the hormone of the medulla in organic solvents, and this finding was utilized later when a method for extraction of hormones of the cortex was devised.

During the exploratory stage of a project in biochemistry the appearance of a precipitate or a change in color or the presence of an odor may be the turning point that leads to success. It is a matter of some comfort and reassurance if more than one of these little indicators are available for examination. It is like having money in a savings bank.

The second straw in the wind was an odor. Adrenal glands themselves have an unusual, pleasant, butterlike odor that is persistent. In the search for a method of isolation for the hormone, adrenal glands were treated with acetone, methanol, ethanol, isopropanol, and benzene; the extracts were then separated from the meaty residue and concentrated. The odor originally contained in the gland persisted in these extracts. It was volatile either in a partial vacuum or at atmospheric pressure.

53

It seemed possible that the odor was a decomposition product of the hormone. If the structure of the odor could be determined, this might be a first step in identification of the desired product. A volatile compound was isolated, a derivative was made, and analysis revealed its structure. The odor did not come from the adrenal cortex but was an impurity in the benzene that had been used to extract the gland. This experience resulted in a rigid rule of procedure: never use benzene of any commercial grade without purifying it with concentrated sulfuric acid. Since 1933 this simple laboratory rule has avoided many a headache and much waste of time.

The compound that was isolated obviously did not explain the odor of the adrenal cortex, and in twenty-five years no progress has been made in this aspect of the investigation.

As the financial depression began to lift, it became possible to add Mayo Foundation Fellows for work in biochemistry. Seldom do such Fellows make outstanding contributions during the relatively short sojourn in the laboratory. However, Dr. Giles A. Koelsche carried out a project concerned with the relationship between the thyroid and the adrenal glands. Although he was not familiar with laboratory procedures, his great interest in the problem and his determination to make the work a success resulted in a thesis which was accepted. He was awarded the degree of doctor of philosophy in medicine.

Four additions to the personnel of the laboratory during 1933 and 1934 were of first importance. William D. Allers was appointed to succeed Dr. Koelsche; Szent-Györgyi's assistant Dr. Svirbely was added to the staff for one year; Warren F. McGuckin and Miss Helen M. Cassidy began their association with the laboratory.

Allers was the first to show that adrenalectomized dogs could be maintained indefinitely, without a trace of the extract of the adrenal cortex, provided that sodium chloride and a basic sodium salt, such as citrate, were added to the diet. Dr. George Harrop had demonstrated this possibility but in his dogs the concentration of potassium in the blood was above normal and he occasionally found it necessary to give small amounts of adrenal cortical extract to maintain the mineral salts of the blood within normal limits.

Allers went further and showed that, with a diet low in potassium but with a high intake of sodium chloride and sodium citrate, no extract of the adrenal cortex was necessary and the electrolytes in the blood remained within normal limits indefinitely.

Dr. Svirbely's previous work with Professor King at Pittsburgh and with Dr. Szent-Györgyi at Szeged had already been mentioned. He was well prepared to carry out a project concerning the influence of vitamin C on the symptoms of adrenal deficiency in the dog and the influence of the hormones of the adrenal cortex on scurvy in the guinea pig. This was original work. No investigator in the field of scurvy had had hormones of the adrenal cortex available, and no one who worked with adrenalectomized dogs had studied the effect of vitamin C on these animals. Svirbely showed that in dogs vitamin C cannot act vicariously for the hormones of the adrenal cortex after adrenalectomy. An extract of the adrenal cortex does modify the symptoms of scurvy but cannot maintain guinea pigs on a scorbutic diet. Adrenalectomy does not alter the ability of the dog to make vitamin C when the animal subsists on a scorbutic diet.

Seven

The Quest for "Cortin"

THE YEARS 1930 to 1940 were occupied with the quest for "cortin, the hormone of the adrenal cortex." Progress in the chemical investigation was closely tied to a study of the physiologic activity of this hormone, but as the years passed both aspects of the work became more and more confused.

Cortin (a name for "the hormone" suggested by Hartman and co-workers) was known to be soluble in water and in organic solvents, but each group of workers engaged in research on the adrenal cortex devised its own procedure for its preparation. The extracts varied in the content of cortin, in the amounts of impurities, and in the duration of physiologic activity in the extract.

After three years of trial and error, we isolated a small amount of crystalline material. This marked the end of the first phase of the investigation and opened the doors to new prospects and problems. The next step seemed to be the accumulation of a large amount of the crystals as rapidly as possible, to permit both chemical identification and a study of physiologic activity. In 1934 it seemed probable that cortin would soon take its place beside thyroxin and glutathione. The same pattern of progress appeared to be unfolding; the most tedious part of the work lay behind us; the most interesting part and the solution of the problem apparently were at hand.

The adrenal gland is the source not only of cortin but also of epinephrine, better known as adrenalin. Cortin had been talked about for less than five years, but adrenalin had been an article of commerce for more than thirty years. In 1901 Parke Davis and Co. had trademarked the word "adrenalin," which meant that, while other pharmaceutical companies could separate epinephrine from the adrenal gland or prepare it by synthesis, they could not sell the compound under that name.

The sale of epinephrine under whatever name may seem a digression. However, just as epinephrine is associated closely with the cortical hormones in the adrenal gland, so also epinephrine and the cortical hormones remained intimately related throughout the investigation of the adrenal cortex. In fact, recovery of epinephrine afforded an unlimited supply of adrenal glands.

From a chemical standpoint, it is possible to separate both epinephrine and cortin from the same sample of glands, but up to 1934 no pharmaceutical company had done this. At that time Parke Davis supplied almost all the epinephrine sold through retail drugstores in the United States. Epinephrine sold under the name adrenalin was in strong demand; sold under any other name it was a "drug on the market." This explains why Parke Davis was interested in adrenal glands, and also why no other pharmaceutical company was.

From the beginning of our chemical investigation McKenzie and I were mindful of the economic advantage that would accrue from utilization of both epinephrine and cortin from adrenal glands, and in 1934 we believed that our method would permit such a procedure. With this possibility in mind, I approached the president of Parke Davis.

Our proposal was that the company should buy bovine adrenal glands and deliver them to the Mayo Foundation in Rochester free of charge. In return, we would separate both cortin and epinephrine, retain the cortical extract for our own use, and send the epinephrine to Parke Davis in Detroit. In that way we would receive glands free of charge and Parke Davis would receive adrenalin without cost of labor.

There was one detail of this arrangement that could be regarded as a hazard, or joker. We agreed unconditionally to deliver to Parke Davis the same amount of adrenalin that would have been separated in the firm's own laboratories from the glands that we received.

With more hope than assurance, that contract was signed in 1934. It was terminated in 1949. The total weight of glands that we treated was 150 tons. The epinephrine that we delivered was of little value to us but was worth more than $9 million when sold as adrenalin in retail stores.

The average amount of epinephrine separated from bovine adrenal glands by the Parke Davis laboratories was 0.165 percent of the weight of the glands. Whatever doubts McKenzie and I had that we would not be able to match the stipulated yield were set at rest by another agreement with Wilson Laboratories, wholly owned subsidiary of the Wilson Packing Co., Chicago, Illinois. Wilson Laboratories had devised a method for the preparation of an extract of the adrenal cortex and were equipped with apparatus with which to make it, but they did not have facilities for biologic standardization of cortin.

Dr. David Klein, president of Wilson Laboratories, agreed to give to the Mayo Foundation 300 pounds of bovine adrenal glands each week if we would standardize the cortical extract prepared in their laboratories. Furthermore, we would be allowed to keep all the epinephrine that was separated from the glands. With this as a reserve, so to speak, we believed we could meet the terms of the contract with Parke Davis. This contract was to provide 600 pounds of glands a week. This, with the 300 pounds a week from Wilson Laboratories, was a sure source of starting material, but this flood of glandular tissue presented formidable problems. These are described later, but first some aspects of our experience with adrenalin should be recorded here, for they illuminate the slow unfolding of ultimate truth.

The first shipment of adrenalin to Parke Davis was the source of much satisfaction and pride on our part. Some time later we were chagrined to receive a letter stating that the adrenalin contained 5.0 percent mineral matter. This amount was a gross contamination, far more than was permissible. There was only one procedure that could surmount this difficulty: analysis of the ash left after ignition. When this was done it was shown that the ash was magnesium phosphate. McKenzie and I then devised a method for removal of magnesium phosphate without loss of adrenalin. The total ash content was reduced to not more than 0.1 percent. The pure white, ash-free, finely crystalline material, in lots of 300 grams, was hermetically sealed in an atmosphere of nitrogen in Pyrex flasks. Prepared in this manner, the adrenalin remained colorless indefinitely. Again we felt justifiable pride in the achievement.

Some years later an officer of Parke Davis and Co. visited our laboratory, and I pointed out to him a large glass jar containing a thick layer of freshly precipitated adrenalin. When he saw this, he remarked, "Do you know there is a tradition that we cannot make pure adrenalin in our laboratory but that you can?" To my certain knowledge this tradition ceased to exist many years ago.

Our fears about meeting the terms of our contract quickly disappeared, never to return. At first there was a small deficiency in the weekly yield, which was brought up to the required weight with epinephrine from the glands sent by Wilson Laboratories, but as experience was gained, the yields rose above 0.165 percent and sometimes were as high as 0.250. All in excess of 0.165 percent was retained by us and was sold on the market.

In 1934 the price of bovine adrenal glands was 20 cents a pound. As the use of cortical extract increased, the supply of glands in respect to demand became more and more limited, and finally the price reached the fantastic figure of $3.00 a pound. The total cost of the glands processed in our laboratory was close to $200,000. This formidable sum was eliminated from our budget by the "intimate relation between adrenalin and the cortical hormones."

It is necessary to close this disgression about adrenalin on an ironic note. In 1949, forty-eight years after the discovery of adrenalin, Tullar* found that the adrenal medulla produces a second active substance that is closely related to adrenalin.

Thus, all the adrenalin that we had sent to Parke Davis and Co. contained from 10 to 20 percent of this other hormone, norepinephrine. Both of these compounds are in the adrenal medulla; both are soluble in dilute acids and are precipitated by ammonium hydroxide. Both were in our "pure white, ash-free, finely crystalline material."

In his memoirs Dr. Russell M. Wilder, discussing a patient who

* B. F. Tullar, *Science,* 109:536-7 (1949).

had paroxysmal hypertension that appeared to be caused by pheo-chromocytoma, says, ". . . the diabetic service was called in consultation because sugar had been found in the urine. . . . I was in attendance at the operation and was able to secure half the tumor. I took this personally to Dr. Edward C. Kendall. . . . I recall my excitement when two days later . . . he handed me a small test tube one-quarter full of white crystalline epinephrine."*

Since we had a method for separation of epinephrine from adrenal glands, it was not difficult to treat the adrenomedullary tumor in a similar manner, and a large amount of epinephrine was separated. However, this was not the last of this incident. Some years later Professor Otto Krayer, of the Harvard Medical School, asked me whether the epinephrine separated from this tumor contained norepinephrine. Judging from work carried out later by Goldenberg, Chargaff, and associates, probably from 50 to 90 percent of the "adrenalin" was, in fact, norepinephrine.

Adrenal glands are reddish brown, and after they have been passed through a meat grinder they resemble ground round steak. About 80 percent of the weight is water. The first problem was to separate the aqueous phase from the protein and fat. For almost five years acetone was employed for this purpose. We then found that ethyl alcohol possessed many advantages. The desired compounds were in the aqueous phase, and after extraction with 85 percent alcohol, the "meaty" residue and fat did not contain more of the cortin that would be present in the water that could not be pressed out. The same relationship was true for the distribution of epinephrine. McKenzie pointed out that a second extraction of the meaty residue with alcohol would not be justified by the yield. The decision not to re-extract the residue, after the initial aqueous phase had been pressed out, was wise and timely. We were confronted with many problems concerned with the "assembly line" type of preparation of cortical extract. To have complicated this with extra work that could not yield a significant increase in either cortical or medullary hormones would have been an error.

The necessity to secure the maximal yield of epinephrine had a

* *Perspectives in Biology and Medicine,* 1:253 (1958).

strong influence on the development of the method for extraction. For example, we knew that ferric salts destroy epinephrine and also produce a dark color. Since we wanted a pure-white epinephrine we removed traces of iron with ferrocyanide ion.

Furthermore, the epinephrine was protected by the addition of sulfurous acid (SO_2 in ethanol). This antioxidant preserved the epinephrine while it was in aqueous solution. The alcohol and most of the water were removed with water-pump suction at a temperature not above 20 degrees C. in a series of six 22-liter flasks. The flasks were connected with six galvanized-iron condensers, one for each flask. These metal receivers were made by welding together the top and bottom portions of discarded 30-gallon hot-water tanks after removal of the middle section. A large refrigeration unit was installed to maintain the cooling bath around the condensers at −10 degrees C.

The process began on Saturday morning. The glands, in a frozen state, were ground, added to ice-cold ethanol, 85 percent, and placed in the cold room. On Monday morning the aqueous-alcoholic phase was pressed from the "meaty" residue. During Monday, Tuesday, Wednesday, and on Thursday morning, the alcohol was removed and the water was concentrated. On Friday the concentrated aqueous solution was extracted with chloroform. The chloroform solution of the cortin was concentrated, and the cortin again was dissolved in water. This aqueous solution, freed of traces of chloroform, contained all of the cortical activity of the adrenal glands. Saturday morning the whole cycle started over again. We did not enlarge the laboratory space, but we multiplied the assistants by three and ran the process with three 8-hour shifts for 24 hours a day.

From a psychological standpoint, this was a stimulating program. The constant rushing sound from six water-suction pumps plus the refrigeration unit imparted a sense of power and urgency. One visitor who stood in the midst of the assembly remarked, "I feel as though the work was rushing along at sixty miles an hour." This pilot-plant factory continued, not for weeks or months, but for thirteen years. The hormones were produced in a steady flow.

Separation of epinephrine exerted a most important influence on the investigation. Epinephrine is affected by light, heat, and traces of catalysts that assist oxidation. Throughout the interval in which the method of preparation of an extract was developed, the preservation of epinephrine was uppermost in our minds. This was necessary: we had signed a contract to deliver the epinephrine. But, in a chemical sense, what was good for epinephrine was good for cortin. The end result was that epinephrine became one of the major factors in the chemical investigation.

Throughout the entire time of preparation of the extract, slight changes were made whenever they were found to be desirable. Substitution of ethanol for acetone has been mentioned. Benzene was used at first to extract the aqueous solution. This was changed to chloroform. For some years the first steps were carried out at room temperature. Subsequently they were performed at 0 degrees C. All traces of lecithin were removed, since lecithin, in turn, permitted small amounts of epinephrine to pass into the chloroform. Finally, if the concentrated aqueous solution was allowed to stand at 0 degrees for 18 hours (overnight), some insoluble material slowly separated. The opalescent turbidity was a source of irritation for months, until it was found that barium ion, precipitated with sulfate, would completely remove this impurity.

Until biologic methods of standardization were established, it was not possible to manufacture, on a commercial scale, an extract of the adrenal cortex that would have a constant potency. The extracts were prepared from the same weight of glands, and this was about all that could be done at the time. All pharmaceutical companies exercised meticulous care and used any information at hand, to provide a measure of potency for cortical adrenal extracts. Some employed as a criterion the rate of growth of adrenalectomized rats. Others used the amount of extract needed to maintain adrenalectomized dogs. Large sums of money were expended, but for many years the situation was confused.

In 1934 it appeared that the only satisfactory answer to this situation was isolation of cortin in the form of a pure substance. We believed that our highly refined aqueous extract of the adrenal cortex would provide that answer.

To start with material that resembles hamburger and to separate a few milligrams of crystalline material is similar to bringing a pearl of great beauty from the murky depths of the sea. As a gland of internal secretion the adrenal cortex is a marvelous machine.

63

Anatomists and physiologists have studied the performance of this gland and defined its function in broad terms, but these disciplines cannot go beyond certain fixed limits. The full explanation of how the gland performs its function must await the work of the chemist. Hence, with full realization that a rare opportunity was at hand, H. L. Mason, C. S. Myers, B. F. McKenzie, and I accepted the task before us. A steady supply of the extract was available and we soon were able to devise a method of fractionation that was effective.

The aqueous extract of the adrenal cortex was extracted with benzene until all physiologic activity had been taken into this solvent. Some inert material remained in the aqueous phase. This was designated "aqueous residue." The benzene was concentrated to a volume convenient to use and was in turn extracted with water as long as active material passed from the benzene into the aqueous phase. A large amount of the total extractive remained in the benzene. This portion was designated "benzene residue." The water extract was concentrated to a convenient volume and extracted again with benzene. The alternate distribution between water and benzene was repeated many times, and gradually the material originally soluble in water was separated into three fractions: those compounds more soluble in benzene than in water—that is, the combined benzene residues; those components more soluble in water than in benzene— that is, the combined aqueous residues; and the material that passed freely from water into benzene and then was extracted from benzene with water.

Removal of benzene from the first fraction and treatment of the residue with water and other solvents afforded crystalline compounds A and B. From the second fraction it was not difficult to crystallize compounds C and D, and from the third fraction compound E was crystallized from ethanol. Several other compounds were subsequently separated from each fraction, but those closely resembled the other members of the groups to which they belonged.

Those were exciting days. It was becoming apparent that we had to deal not only with "the hormone" of the adrenal cortex but with a large group of compounds that were closely related. Which of them would prove to be cortin?

The identification of a hitherto unknown organic compound requires analysis to determine the different elements in the compound and the amount of each element present. The molecular weight also must be determined. Then the empirical formula can be established. The formulation of the architecture or arrangement of the atoms requires a study of the chemical properties of the compound and the preparation of derivatives and degradation products. A few years before 1930 this work could not have been carried out unless a large amount of material was available. Fortunately for us, the technique of microanalysis had been developed by Professor Pregal and others, and all the required analyses could be performed with only a few milligrams. As the number of crystalline compounds from the extract increased, we realized that many analyses would be required.

The first few samples were sent out of the laboratory for analysis, but some of the reports that we received were not correct. We were eager to get on with the work; delay was a source of frustration and irritation. The best remedy for this situation was to buy the necessary equipment and make the analyses in our own laboratory.

A microanalytic balance and all the special apparatus were purchased; Dr. Mason assumed the heavy responsibility of microanalyst; and we soon were independent of outside help. The results of the analyses were always reliable and the work progressed smoothly.

Research in any institution is influenced directly and indirectly by the nature of that institution. The laboratory in the Mayo Foundation was fortunate because of the widespread interest in the adrenal cortex. Internist and surgeon, pathologist and physiologist, each had something to contribute.

An important new factor in the physiologic work was introduced in September 1934 when Dwight Ingle was added to the staff. He was endowed with an insatiable urge to find out why certain things are so. One of these things was concerned with the endocrine glands. What did the endocrine glands have to do with contraction of muscle? He had taken every course in psychology at the University of Idaho and, still in search of an answer, had taken graduate courses in the department of psychology at the University of Minnesota.

Earlier in 1934 a paper was published by W. T. Heron, W. M. Hales, and D. J. Ingle; I am quite sure that Ingle was the one most involved in its preparation. The paper described a new apparatus for recording the response of muscle to faradic stimulation. Work was performed by contraction of the muscle; the amount of work was recorded on a cyclometer. Rats were anesthetized and fixed to a board, and the Achilles tendon was attached to a 100-gram weight. The muscle was stimulated three times each second as long as the rat continued to respond. If given repeated doses of the anesthetic agent, water and glucose, the normal rat would respond for 10 or 12 days. After adrenalectomy, rats treated in the same manner ceased to respond in less than 24 hours. This apparatus could be used to explore many problems in physiology. However, it has not been widely adopted, for one good reason: there was always the question of which would fail first, the rat or the operator of the machine.

In 1934, when Dwight asked me whether I was interested in the standardization of cortical extracts, the most important problem concerned with the physiologic aspects of the investigation seemed on the way to an answer. His appointment was one of the turning points of the investigation.

From the start of our investigation of the adrenal cortex, maintenance of adrenalectomized dogs had been the basis for standardization of extracts. This method also was used for assay of the samples of extracts that were made in the Wilson Laboratories.

The method was reliable, provided certain factors were controlled. These factors were the responsiveness of each individual dog; the diet; and the daily intake of sodium, potassium, and chloride. If the dog was not sensitive to lack of cortical extract, that animal would survive an "adrenal crisis" far better than would a dog that was hypersensitive. If the condition of each dog was not checked at frequent intervals during the day, an adrenal crisis could develop quite rapidly and the sensitive animal would be found dead. It is obvious that after some months those dogs that were hypersensitive would have died and only the nonsensitive dogs would be left. Such a colony of animals could not provide results that could be compared with those from another group in which insensitive dogs were eliminated as soon as their lack of response was recognized.

Diet of the dogs was important. If thrice-boiled lean meat was fed and the water was discarded, the high-protein and low-sodium intake would cause a rapid increase in blood urea (300 milligrams or more per 100 milliliters of blood) within two or three days. With use of low-protein, high-salt intake, the blood urea would remain low for many days.

The daily intake of mineral salts was even more important. An intake high in sodium and low in potassium maintained the dogs without the need for any extract whatever. With a high-potassium and low-sodium intake it was difficult to maintain them, even with large amounts of extract.

The factors of responsiveness, diet, and intake of minerals were encountered in all laboratories, but each group of investigators developed its own rules of standardization. This situation caused some anxious moments in our laboratory. Swingle and Pfiffner at Princeton University employed adrenalectomized dogs for standardization of cortical adrenal extracts, and stated that there were 2000 dog units in 1 kilogram of bovine adrenal glands. Under the conditions that were used in our laboratory, we found that 1 kilogram of bovine adrenal glands contained 200 dog units. This discrepancy of 1000 percent was too great to be disregarded. It could be caused in two ways. Either our method, although apparently satisfactory, extracted only 10 percent as much cortin as did the Princeton method or, if our extract was as good as that of Swingle and Pfiffner, the standard dog unit in Rochester, Minnesota, must be ten times that in Princeton.

Samples of extracts were exchanged between the two laboratories, and the second explanation was soon found to be the correct one, but this incident shows in what a confused state was the standardization of extracts of the adrenal cortex.

Adrenalectomized dogs maintained with an extract of the adrenal cortex or with the necessary intake of mineral salts can be used to secure physiologic results that can be tabulated and subjected to statistical analysis. In this respect, the physiologic results resemble the results of chemical analyses. However, adrenalectomized dogs are not chemical reagents, and something more is needed than a janitor to dust them off now and then.

The value of a colony of adrenalectomized dogs is determined by the care that they receive. The steady accumulation of data concerning physiologic activity that came from our colony of dogs was made possible by the high quality of attention given by the man who watched over them. Regardless of social or other engagements, whether or not he himself was ill disposed, Donald Krockow was at the side of the sick animal day and night as long as it was necessary.

Don joined our group in December 1935, to replace Mr. Allers. He was a graduate of St. Olaf College, Northfield, Minnesota. Although he did not have a medical degree, he had the sterling characteristics of a general practitioner devoted to the health and happiness of his patients. His name will recur often.

In the fall of 1935 Dr. Hugo W. Nilson came to our laboratory to carry out an extension of the investigation of mineral metabolism in adrenalectomized dogs. He rounded out the work of Allers and gathered convincing evidence that potassium could cause the distressing symptoms associated with deficiency of the adrenal cortex. Nilson's work involved many analyses of sodium, chloride, and potassium. Miss Eva Hartzler was added to the staff to handle these.

In 1936 Willard Hoehn joined the laboratory. Hoehn had just acquired the degree of doctor of philosophy in chemistry from Iowa State University.

Shortly after the demonstration of the presence of a hormone of the adrenal cortex by Swingle and Pfiffner at Princeton University, the department of biochemistry at Columbia University decided to carry on work in this field. Dr. Pfiffner and Dr. Oskar Wintersteiner were given appointments to investigate the chemistry of the adrenal cortex. This was a strong combination. The former had published a method for extraction of cortin, and the latter was a chemist of recognized ability as an analyst and investigator in organic chemistry. The results of their study were presented at the annual meetings of the Federation of American Societies for Experimental Biology in 1934 and 1935. We knew of their progress and of their conclusions about the chemical nature of cortin, but we believed that the broad foundation that had been built to support the work in our laboratory justified continuation of our project. On the other hand, they had faith in their approach and decided to continue the investigation at Columbia.

This situation was disturbed in 1936 by publication of seven papers that dealt with the chemistry of the adrenal cortex. These papers, written by Professor Tadeus Reichstein and his associates of the Technische Hochschule in Zürich, Switzerland, showed that Professor Reichstein was well on his way toward the heart of the problem. We had reported the isolation of five crystalline compounds. Pfiffner and Wintersteiner also had described the isolation of five compounds. But Reichstein now reported the separation of seven substances. In each laboratory the first crystalline compound to be isolated was designated A, the second one B, and so on, down the alphabet. Comparison of samples of compound A from the three laboratories showed them to be quite different, and this was true also of all the rest. On the basis of a description of the chemical properties, such as melting points and specific rotation, it became clear that our compound E was compound F of Pfiffner and compound Fa of Reichstein and his associates.

It is unfortunate that steps were not taken immediately to arrange a uniform nomenclature. The order could then easily have been changed, thus simplifying the publication of papers concerned with the adrenal cortex. For example, many years after these early papers, other authors would refer in the same publication to compounds E, F, and S. The first two, E and F, were ours, since Reichstein's compounds E and F were inactive. The S represented one of Reichstein's, since our series did not include S.

Publication of the seven papers by Reichstein and his associates was interpreted by the group at Columbia University as evidence that the point of diminishing returns in this field had been reached. Dr. Pfiffner accepted a position in the laboratory of Parke Davis and Co., and Dr. Wintersteiner went to the laboratory of E. R. Squibb and Sons at New Brunswick, New Jersey. The former made several contributions concerned with the isolation and chemistry of folic acid. The latter was the first to crystallize penicillin and has made many contributions in the fields of antibiotic agents, hormones, and the structure of natural products.

In 1937 Reichstein published another paper, in which he described the isolation and properties of his group's substance H. In the laboratory of Professor Ernst Laqueur in Amsterdam, Holland, substance H was found to be by far the most active product isolated in Reichstein's laboratory in Zürich. On the basis of these pharmacologic tests, substance H was believed to be the long-sought hormone cortin; it was given the place of honor and designated "corticosterone."

When the 1937 paper reached our laboratory, we too were faced with an important decision. Had the time arrived to withdraw from the formidable competition offered by Reichstein's group, or should we continue? In the field of organic chemistry we were at a great disadvantage, since the experience and outstanding ability of Professor Reichstein would enable him to identify and perhaps to synthesize the crystalline compounds in the adrenal cortex far more rapidly than we could.

Nevertheless, the papers of the Zürich group had not cut the ground from under our feet.

The project was not yet limited to organic chemistry. Cortin had not been identified, and until this had been accomplished the door was still open. Moreover, we possessed two advantages. The first was a large, steady supply of adrenal extract. Frozen adrenal glands were delivered to our door every week and would continue to be because the epinephrine from these glands was being shipped to Detroit according to schedule. On the other hand, the adrenal extract available to Professor Reichstein was not only limited in comparison, but the continuity of the supply was doubtful. The Zürich investigators did not make their own extractions from the adrenal cortex; this was done by Organon, Inc., a pharmaceutical manufacturing company in Oss, Holland. The president of the company, Dr. Zwanenberg, had visited me in 1936. He told me that several $10,000 batches of extract had been sent to Zürich, but he also intimated that progress had been slow and that if something did not happen soon, his company might tire of the arrangement.

Our second advantage lay in the physiologic work we had done. The experiments of Dwight Ingle and Donald Krockow provided a constant flow of reliable data. I was in daily contact with this vital part of the investigation. In the quest for cortin all fractions were carefully examined. Experimental work such as that of Allers, Nilson, and Ingle on the influence of mineral salts on cortical adrenal deficiency also contributed to our background information. Additional stimulus and satisfaction came from the use of our extract in the treatment of patients at the Mayo Clinic. Professor Reichstein was remote from all these aspects of the search.

Laqueur, who was professor of pharmacology in the University of Amsterdam, Holland, was much interested in the endocrine glands and had published books and many papers in this field. Testosterone had been isolated and named in his laboratory. Professor Laqueur was also a director of Organon, Inc., and for that reason was familiar with the preparation of the extract of the adrenal glands made for Professor Reichstein. He agreed to assay the extracts in his laboratory at the university. Three methods were employed: the muscle-twitch test of Everse and de Fremery; a test based on the ability of a rat to swim; and a limited assay by means of adrenalectomized dogs. The method of Everse and de Fremery, which required only a few minutes, was quite different from that used by Ingle. In the adrenalectomized rat an extract of the adrenal cortex did modify the response of the muscle to stimulation, but the significance of this was not at all clear and could not be related to other physiologic processes. This test of the potency of cortical adrenal extracts was not long in favor. The swimming test with rats also was a crude measure of potency.

For various reasons, then, we were not dismayed by the suggestion that substance H of Reichstein's group was cortin. Substance H was our compound B, which had been isolated two years before. We had shown that it had a marked influence on the capacity of muscle to perform work, but that its effect on mineral metabolism was slight. We were certain that this substance could not be cortin. The decision at the Mayo Foundation was to continue investigation of the adrenal cortex.

Eight

Cortin Is a Steroid

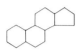

DURING 1936 FIVE different aspects of this investigation had been carried on with all possible vigor. These were: isolation of cortin and related substances; investigation of the chemical nature of cortin; standardization of cortin; study of the physiologic significance of cortin; and clinical use of cortin.

As a product of the first aspect of the research, a paper was published that showed that although our compound E, previously mentioned, did not possess androgenic properties, it could be converted into a "diketone" that had from one-fourth to one-sixth the androgenic activity of androstenedione. Compound E had already been shown to have the qualitative properties of cortin, and the transformation of E into an androgen definitely linked cortin with the structure of the steroids. This was the first published evidence that cortin was a steroid. If this was so, then all the other crystalline compounds closely related to compound E were members of the same family.

Reichstein had published a paper that showed that adrenosterone, which was one of the first compounds separated in his series, was an androgen. He also had found that another compound separated from the gland could be degraded to a ketone that was an androgen. However, none of the compounds used by Reichstein possessed the properties of cortin. This was strong presumptive

73

evidence for the presence of the steroid-ring system, but it did not furnish evidence that would link cortin with that family of compounds.

The paper that contained our results was published in the issue of the *Journal of Biological Chemistry* for November 1936. The title was "The Identification of a Substance Which Possesses the Qualitative Action of Cortin: Its Conversion into a Diketone Closely Related to Androstenedione." Readers of that conservative journal must have been confused to discover another paper in the same issue with the title "Chemical Studies on the Adrenal Cortex. Isolation of Two New Physiologically Inactive Compounds." The authors were Oskar Wintersteiner and J. J. Pfiffner. Although there was a flat contradiction in the two titles, the two papers concerned the same substance, which was compound E in our series and compound F in theirs. There is a simple explanation for the contradiction. We used the method of Ingle, which measured the capacity of muscle to perform work; they used as a measure the influence of the compound upon mineral metabolism. We had also tried that method of assay and had found but slight effect. For that reason the words "qualitative action of cortin" were used in our title.

The word cortin carried an aura of glamour. It designated the compound that possessed the highest potency for maintenance of weight, strength, and well-being. In addition to causing these effects, the compound, in a daily dose of a small fraction of a milligram, was believed to be able to control the concentration of urea and the mineral constituents in the blood.

There were two reasons why belief in the unitary nature of cortin was so widespread and so firmly fixed. The first was the result of the original concept that "the hormone" of an endocrine gland must possess the physiologic properties of an extract of that gland. After that idea had been fixed in the minds of biologists, physiologists, biochemists, and clinicians, it became deep-rooted and immovable. The second reason was that the only method of assay for the active crystalline compounds separated from the adrenal cortex was the one devised by Dwight Ingle and used in our laboratory. No other laboratory had adopted the method, and perhaps it was just as well. Within a short period Dwight had determined the relative activity of all the crystalline compounds that were available. What was then needed was an independent criterion that could be used to prove or disprove these results.

Such information eventually was found in abundance, but the pathway of those who brought it was rough and devious.

In financial circles the statement is sometimes made that "the market closed on a firm note." So it was with us. We had met a crisis and had survived.

It is no longer necessary to detail the progress of the chemical investigation of the adrenal cortex. The scientific world now knows that all the crystalline compounds separated from the adrenal gland were completely identified. So many years after the event it matters little whether the most significant contributions came from Zürich, Switzerland, or Rochester, Minnesota, U. S. A. The honors were divided. Neither group discovered all the pertinent facts. The important thing is that the work was completed.

The uninitiated might infer that, with acquisition and identification of the crystalline compounds, it would be a relatively short and easy task to show what physiologic processes were influenced and what chemical reactions were modified. During 1937 and 1938 progress with these problems was made in our laboratory, but this pertained to the nature of cortin rather than to the mode of action of the compound.

Corticosterone (Reichstein's substance H and our compound B) was studied from a quantitative standpoint. The finding was that 1.5 milligram of B was required as a daily dose for an adrenalectomized dog weighing 13.0 kilograms; 1 milligram was not adequate. The conclusion was drawn that corticosterone possessed all the qualitative properties of cortin and that therefore cortin presumably was closely related to corticosterone.

Toward the end of 1937 we found that the material left in solution after separation of compounds A, B, E, and F contained no less than 90 percent of the original activity when this activity was measured by maintenance of adrenalectomized dogs. Last, we had shown that none of the crystalline compounds or any combination of them could be regarded as cortin. The challenge to separate cortin still beckoned us on.

A new departure in the chemical investigation was introduced

75

in 1937. Harold Mason and Willard Hoehn started on an excursion into the field of synthetic organic chemistry to establish the structure of compounds A and B. This involved the conversion of an abundant substance—one of the bile acids—into a degradation product of compound A. The project, which was suggested by Mason, appeared to be of small scope and we hoped to complete it within a short time. I remember how impatient we were over the delay before the sample of desoxycholic acid was received and how eagerly the work was initiated after the sample arrived. The work was actually completed almost a year later.

This was the first synthetic work that concerned the position of the so-called inert or unreactive atom of oxygen. The results taken together with the contribution of R. Tschesche and K. Bohle on sarmentogenin, another steroid that had been isolated from a seed found in Africa, furnished evidence that the atom of oxygen was on carbon 11. May I suggest that my readers reread the preceding sentence and hold in mind carbon 11 of the steroid nucleus? That carbon atom will continue to grow in importance, for it held the clue to the true nature of cortin.

Three other contributions came out of the work in 1937. The first was Ingle's demonstration that the administration of compounds A and B, as well as of the whole extract of the adrenal gland, brought about severe atrophy of the thymus and adrenal glands in normal rats. We had observed that the thymus gland of adrenalectomized dogs hypertrophied in a remarkable manner if the animals were maintained on salts without the aid of cortical extract. Ingle showed that the administration of compounds A and B had the reverse effect. This was useful information concerning the steroids of the adrenal cortex because it was the first work that corroborated and extended Ingle's observations on the influence of compounds A, B, and E on the performance of muscle.

The second contribution came from the Section of Biochemistry and one of the sections of medicine. The work of Allers, Nilson, and Ingle had shown beyond question that the daily intake of potassium is one of the most important factors concerned with the survival and state of well-being in adrenalectomized dogs. Drs. Russell Wilder, Albert Snell, Edwin Kepler, and Edward Rynearson decided to determine whether potassium has an influence on the subjective and objective symptoms of patients with Addison's disease. The results obtained with animals were strikingly duplicated in the patients, with the advantage that the latter could describe their subjective symptoms. For some time patients who had Addison's disease had received much benefit from control of the intake of sodium chloride and sodium citrate. This work proved that it is also necessary to control the amount of potassium in the daily diet.

Four grams of potassium—the amount in a normal daily diet—will promote loss of sodium and chloride. If the intake of potassium were restricted to 1.6 grams, the daily requirement of sodium chloride could be reduced materially. But a daily intake of 1.6 grams of potassium required close supervision and rigid selection of the food that was eaten. Planned diets were included in the paper that was published on this work.

In addition to the four names already mentioned, the paper, when published,* bore the names of Mildred Adams, who was associated with Dr. Power, and myself. We did not realize that the wide publicity given this paper would have an important influence on the next step in the progress of the study of Addison's disease. Neither did we foresee that a special peril was involved with patients maintained for long periods on a diet low in potassium. We did know that adrenalectomized dogs maintained on a low intake of potassium became sensitive to a sudden increase in this element. But the diet of the dogs was kept rigidly constant. When Thanksgiving, Christmas, and New Year's came around, it was difficult for patients to avoid just a bit of turkey or a few extra nuts. Such indulgence could be followed by an acute adrenal crisis and unless cortical extract was available, the patient's life might be forfeited.

The third contribution concerned with physiologic activity was the demonstration that removal of the double bond in the A ring of compounds A and B destroys the physiologic activity. A corresponding double bond is present in testosterone and progesterone, and in these compounds also removal of the bond in the A ring destroys the activity.

What we demonstrated with compounds A and B was to be expected. We were pleased to have been in a position to make the

* Arch. Int. Med., 59:367-393 (1937).

observation. The opportunity was ours because we had accumulated several grams of compounds A and B.

In July 1937 a conference on the adrenal cortex was held at Cold Spring Harbor, New York. For the first three days all the papers concerned the influence of cortin on mineral metabolism. I gave a full summary of our work on the crystalline compounds that we had isolated. C. N. H. Long, R. L. Zwemer, W. W. Swingle, Arthur Grollman, and others emphasized maintenance of animals by control of mineral salts, neglecting the influence of cortin on carbohydrate metabolism. There was but little critical discussion. Everyone was in agreement concerning the most important aspects of the function of cortin.

Almost at the end of the conference however, Dr. S. W. Britton of the University of Virginia presented a paper that dealt with his concept of that function. As early as 1932 he had stated his belief that the "prepotent function" of cortin is concerned with the metabolism of carbohydrates. He had been almost alone in this conclusion then, and at Cold Spring Harbor those present hesitated to accept his viewpoint. Britton had not treated his adrenalectomized animals by control of the mineral metabolism, as others had done. When adrenalectomized animals were given the necessary intake of mineral salts, carbohydrate metabolism could proceed in a normal manner. A high intake of salt was necessary, but even without administration of cortical extract, glycogen was deposited in the liver and muscle, exogenous protein was converted into carbohydrate, and organic metabolism proceeded without interruption. Nevertheless, Britton did show that in an adrenalectomized animal that had been fasted for 18 hours the percentage of glycogen in the liver is close to zero. If an extract of the adrenal cortex is administered during the fast of 18 hours, then glycogen is deposited in the liver. The percentage of glycogen can be increased to normal in this manner.

This observation started a resonance in the attentive mind of Dr. C. N. H. Long. In 1937 Dr. Long was a man with a problem: he could not complete an experiment that was essential to round out some work he had done during the preceding two or three years.

Long and Francis Lukens had made an important contribution to endocrinology that was an extension of the work of Bernardo Houssay in Buenos Aires, Argentina. In an experiment that had brought him world acclaim, Houssay had shown that the state of diabetes and inevitable death that follows the removal of the pancreas could be obviated by removal of the pituitary gland. After both these glands were removed, the animal appeared normal and would live indefinitely. Long and Lukens reported in 1936 that the diabetes is abolished after pancreatectomy, even if the pituitary gland is left intact, provided the adrenal gland is removed. The obvious next experiment to perform was to produce diabetes in such an animal by administration of an extract of the adrenal gland. Long and Lukens had tried to do this, but no effect had been observed.

Although I had not mentioned carbohydrate metabolism in my paper at the conference, later in 1937 Dr. Long asked me for samples of compounds A and B. These were administered to animals in his laboratory, glycosuria was produced, and it immediately became evident that the compounds that brought about this marked effect on carbohydrate metabolism were those that had an atom of oxygen at carbon 11.

Long, Lukens, and others, although primarily interested in diabetes, had thus made an important contribution to understanding of the physiologic activity of cortin. Ingle's observations of the influence of compounds A, B, E, and F on the capacity of muscle to perform work were now matched by the discovery that these same compounds exerted a strong effect on carbohydrate metabolism. This was the beginning of respectability for the carbon 11 group of compounds, A, B, E, and F.

In December 1937 Reichstein wrote to me that he would not be able to continue chemical research on the adrenal cortex, at least for some months. This unexpected information meant that, except for our group, investigation of the nature of cortin had been abandoned. Our determination to continue was unabated. The luster arising from this baffling substance shone with undiminished attraction.

In 1937 M. Steiger and Professor Reichstein had made an outstanding contribution. The first member of the cortical steroids was prepared by alteration of a well-known compound derived from the bile acids. This was the final evidence that cortin belongs to the steroid family. The compound was named desoxycorticosterone.

Professor Reichstein had sent me a sample, and in the summer of 1938 Don Krockow had shown accurately that, measured by the maintenance of adrenalectomized dogs, it was six times as active as corticosterone.

In August 1938 I attended the International Congress of Physiologists in Zürich, where I had the pleasure of meeting Professor Reichstein. He was surprised and happy to hear the report on the activity of his new compound. At the congress he presented a paper that provided the last link required to bring together the synthetic compound and the natural products produced by the gland. He reported isolation of desoxycorticosterone from an extract of the adrenal cortex.

Before this time, by far the largest amount of crystalline material separated from the extract had been prepared in our laboratory. Generous samples of compounds A, B, E, and F had been given to many investigators, but almost all workers believed they were of secondary importance. Cortin, "the hormone" of the adrenal cortex, still held its place as the life-maintaining hormone. Now Reichstein's new crystalline compound, desoxycorticosterone, was available. At the time, it seemed much closer to cortin than anything that had been separated heretofore.

At the Zürich congress I presented the paper that opened the session devoted to the adrenal cortex. Emphasis was placed on the relationship of cortin to mineral metabolism. In 1938 the importance of control of mineral metabolism in adrenalectomized animals was well recognized, and my paper was received without serious criticism. Dr. Hans Selye did not agree that potassium was of great importance, but his remarks were of a general nature and were not supported with experimental results.

Professor Verzar of Budapest gave the other formal paper, which was highly speculative. He had elaborated the hypothesis that cortin was essential in phosphorylation in the body. The experimental work on animals was poorly controlled and the hypothesis was short-lived, but at the end of the discussion he appeared to have convinced the congress that the only important function of the adrenal cortex was concerned with phosphorylation. However, the passage of time has removed those contentions that could not withstand deep probing and has placed a strong foundation under the experimental results that were to endure when carried over to a critical study in the field of clinical medicine.

After the congress I visited Dr. Laqueur in Amsterdam. He had been a guest at our cottage on Lake Zumbro, and his son Peter had worked for some months in my laboratory. Refugees from German universities were coming into Holland in ever-increasing numbers, and Dr. Laqueur was apprehensive of the future. He was an important member of the Dutch organization formed for the relief of German refugees and knew that he would receive special attention from Hitler's storm troopers, but at the dinner table in his home the conversation among his children, then in their late teens and early twenties, was gay. No one could foresee that two daughters and their husbands would become victims of the concentration camp of Bergen-Belsen. They were rescued by the Russians after a year and a half, but one couple died soon after liberation, of spotted fever and hunger edema.

The congress at Zürich was a cross section of physiologists and biochemists throughout the world of science. There was much interest in the adrenal cortex, but the nature of cortin was still a matter of conjecture and there was wide speculation about it. But after the report of the new work by Reichstein it was evident that since desoxycorticosterone had become available it would be possible to answer questions of long standing. For those interested in clinical medicine, the new compound provided the first opportunity to treat patients who had Addison's disease with a substance that was effective and also could be purchased at a price within the reach of most patients.

Dr. George Thorn of the Harvard Medical School assumed leadership of the clinical work. Desoxycorticosterone was administered in all possible ways: by mouth, in the form of pellets placed under the tongue to provide for slow absorption of the compound; by subcutaneous injection; and by implantation of pellets. The pellets were made of the compound alone or were prepared with mixtures of the compound and some inert substance such as cholesterol, that would retard the rate of absorption. Dr. C. F. Code of the Medical School of the University of Minnesota prepared a mixture of desoxycorticosterone and beeswax that was active over long periods.

It soon became apparent that desoxycorticosterone is effective in patients. However, some early observations were not understood. It required some time to relate those untoward results to the true causative factor: mineral metabolism. It should be recalled that the paper from the Mayo Clinic that established the optimal conditions for the treatment of patients who had Addison's disease was published in 1937. The wide publicity given this paper was of benefit to those who were not treated with desoxycorticosterone. It caused the death of many who did receive the new compound.

There were two adverse types of response. In one the blood pressure was increased, edema appeared, the heart became embarrassed, and the patient died of heart failure. In the other, the patients became weak and rapidly lost control of muscular activity to such a degree that they were paralyzed and lay in bed in a helpless and apparently hopeless condition.

Determination of the sodium, potassium, and chloride content in the blood revealed how great was the influence of the new steroid on mineral metabolism. Those who had high blood pressure and edema were found to have high values for sodium and chloride in the blood. Those who were paralyzed had a low concentration of potassium in the blood.

Decrease of the intake of sodium ion relieved the former. Increase in the daily intake of potassium provided a specific and dramatic relief for the latter condition. In other words, a high intake of potassium and a low intake of sodium were required if desoxycorticosterone was administered. This was a complete reversal of the relationships that had been prescribed if desoxycorticosterone was not given to the patient.

The availability of the new steroid for use in clinical medicine and the large number of investigators who became interested assured rapid progress in the study of this first member of the cortical steroids. It was not long before it became evident that the physiologic effects of desoxycorticosterone in patients with Addison's disease closely resemble the influence of mineral salts. Administration of the new compound together with optimal amounts of sodium and potassium ions maintained the concentrations of the mineral constituents of the blood within the normal range, but the patients did not enjoy a sense of well-being; they lost strength and some of them died. This result was very different from that produced in either of the two syndromes that have been described.

If an extract of the adrenal cortex was given, the weakness was relieved and a sense of well-being was restored. This was conclusive evidence that desoxycorticosterone is not "the hormone" of the adrenal cortex. Something more was necessary, and whatever it was, that substance was in the extract of the adrenal cortex.

The physiologic results that came from our laboratory just at this time provided the final evidence that established the true nature of cortin. Many batches of extract, each made from 3,000 pounds of glands, were fractionated and the active material was separated into crystalline steroids and the noncrystalline or amorphous residue. It has already been mentioned that 90 percent of the original activity, in respect to mineral metabolism, was contained in the amorphous fraction. Warren McGuckin was responsible for the treatment of the extract. It was a major contribution and was completed just when the material was most needed.

Dr. Benjamin B. Wells, a Fellow in medicine of the Mayo Foundation, was able to show that the amorphous fraction on a weight basis was from 60 to 100 times more active than corticosterone in its effect on mineral metabolism. It had little effect on carbohydrate metabolism and did not produce atrophy of the thymus and adrenal glands when used in amounts 57 times that which was sufficient to maintain an adrenalectomized dog of 20 kilograms.

These results furnished the clue that had been missing for so long. The unitary nature of cortin had been questioned at frequent intervals, but each time conclusive proof was lacking. The hypothesis that cortin was the steroid that was the most active in both carbohydrate and mineral metabolism had held sway over the minds of most investigators brash enough to express their views in print.

Now two words—"qualitative" and "quantitative"— could be introduced to describe the physiologic action of the crystalline compounds and the amorphous fraction of the adrenal cortex. Those compounds that exerted a qualitative effect on carbohydrate metabolism had but slight influence on mineral metabolism. For the amorphous fraction these relationships were reversed. As soon as it was possible to relate the physiologic effects in quantitative terms, it was obvious that no single crystalline compound or fraction could be regarded as "the hormone" of the adrenal cortex.

At a staff meeting of the Mayo Clinic on May 8, 1940, a paper[*] was read that marked the end of the quest for the individual hormone

---

[*] E. C. Kendall, *Professional Meetings of the Mayo Clinic,* 15:297-304 (1940).

cortin. It contained a statement that represented the consensus of the group who had carried out the work. The adrenal cortex produces a series of compounds that are steroids. Those with oxygen at carbon 11 and an unsaturated ketone in ring A affect carbohydrate metabolism. Compound E is typical of these. Another compound, almost certainly a steroid, which is in the amorphous fraction, has a marked effect on mineral metabolism. Both of these hormones are necessary and sufficient to replace the secretion of the adrenal cortex in the patients with Addison's disease or in adrenalectomized animals.

Ten years after the beginning of the project, the first objective had been reached and the quest for cortin had ended.

A Selection of Photographs

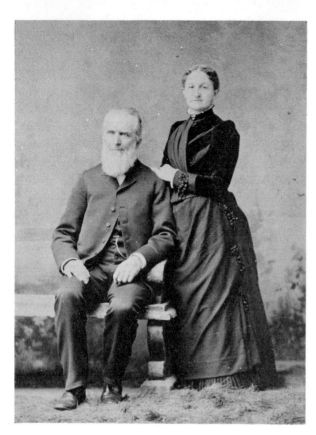

*Grandfather Calvin H.
Kendall and his second
wife, Elena*

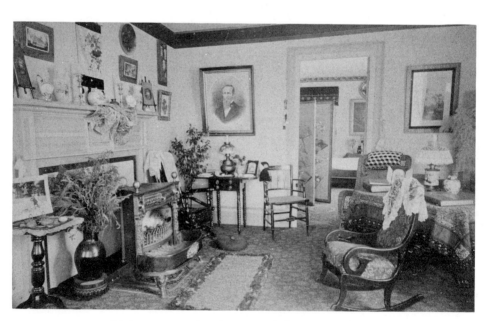

Living room of Calvin Kendall's house, 1890

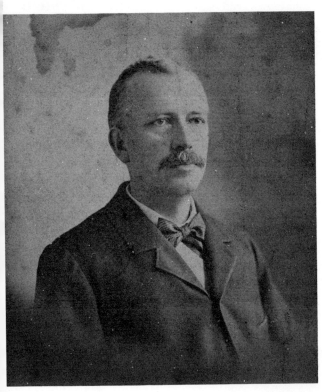

My father, George S. Kendall

My mother, Eva Kendall

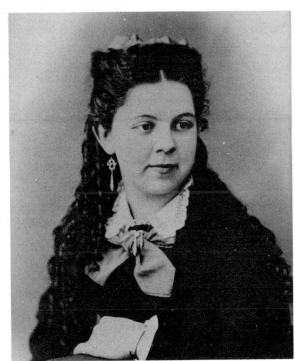

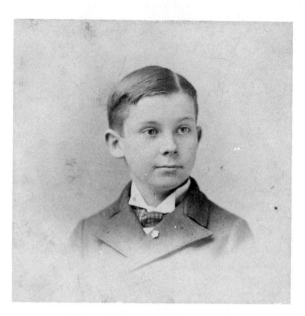

Edward C. Kendall, aged ten

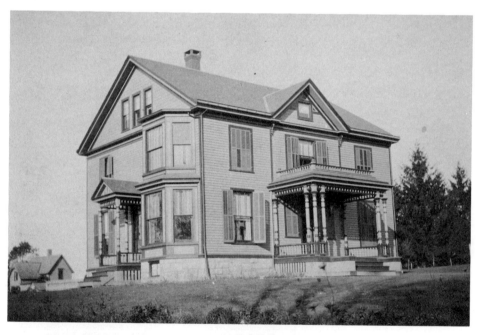

The family home, 51 Elmwood Avenue, South Norwalk, Connecticut

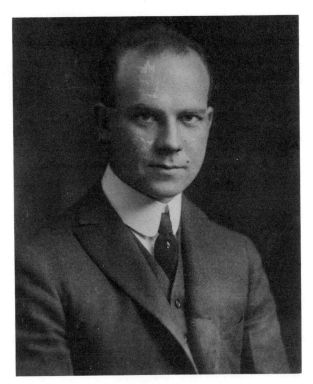

Edward C. Kendall (about 1913)

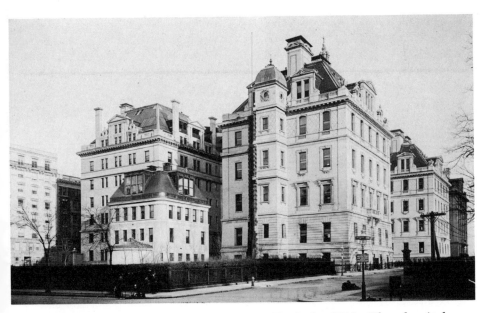

St. Luke's Hospital, New York, New York, in 1913. The chemical laboratory occupied the top floor of the small building in the center

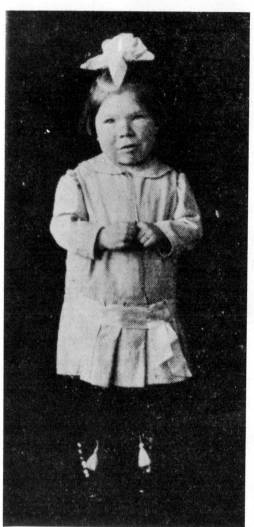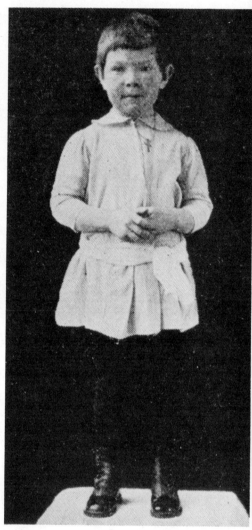

(Left) *A child deficient in thyroid secretion; at age ten her height was 37 inches.* (Right) *The same child after receiving thyroxin for one year; she had grown 6 inches (Mayo Clinic)*

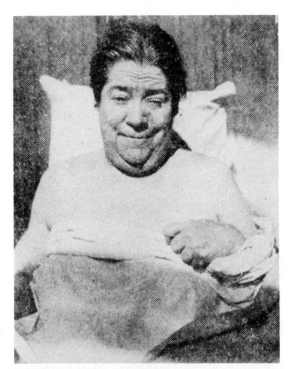

(Above) *A patient deficient in thyroid secretion.* (Below) *The same patient after treatment for a few weeks with partially purified thyroxin (St. Luke's Hospital)*

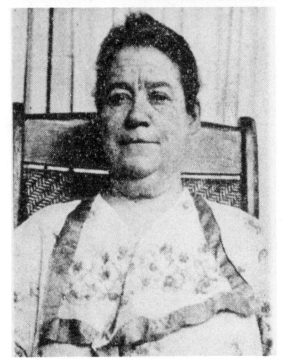

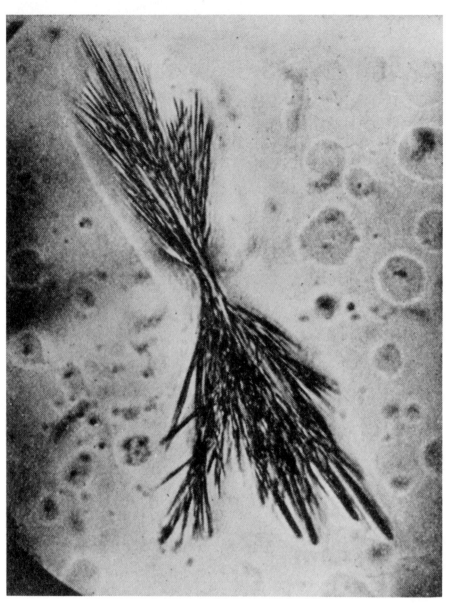

Thyroxin, first crystallized on December 25, 1914 (Mayo Clinic)

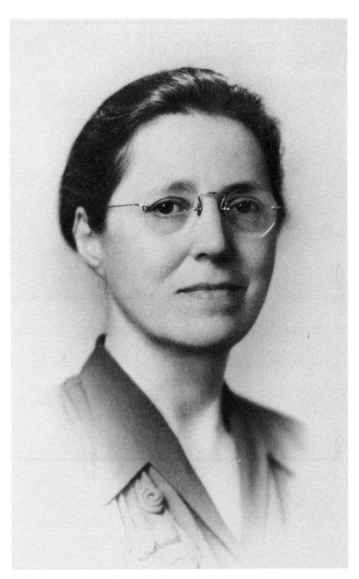

My wife, Rebecca Kendall (about 1940)

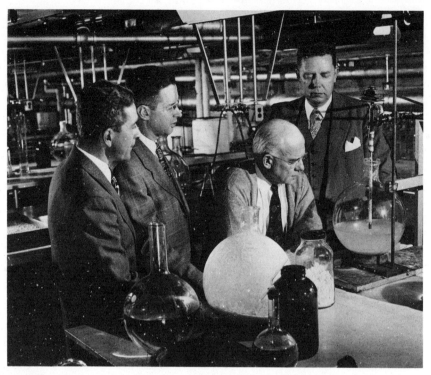

*In the laboratory at the Mayo Clinic after the announcement of the
Nobel Prize, 1950:* (left to right) *Charles H. Slocumb, Howard Polley,
Edward C. Kendall, Philip S. Hench (Mayo Clinic)*

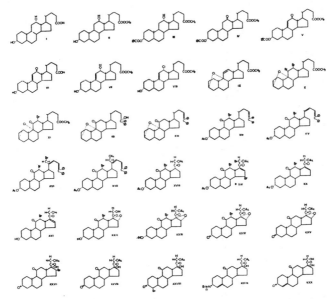

Thirty steps used in the laboratory at the Mayo Clinic for preparation of cortisone from a bile acid (Mayo Clinic)

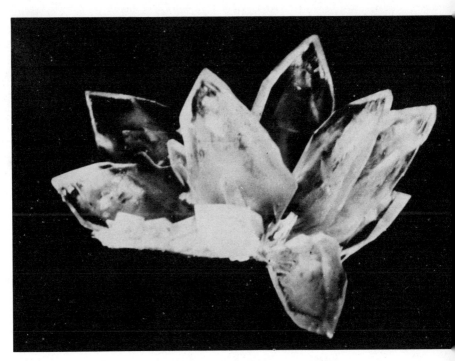

Crystalline cortisone (Mayo Clinic)

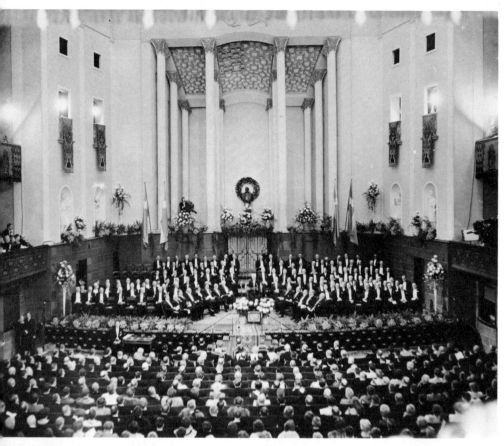

The Nobel Festival, 1950: Convocation in the Concert Hall, Stockholm
(Copyright Reportagebild)

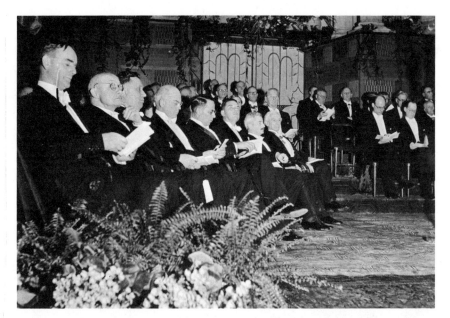

(Front to back) *Nobel laureates Cecil F. Powell (Physics 1950), Otto Diels and Kurt Alder (Chemistry 1950), Edward C. Kendall, Tadeus Reichstein, and Philip S. Hench (Physiology and Medicine 1950), William Faulkner (Literature 1949), and Bertrand Russell (Literature 1950) (Copyright Reportagebild)*

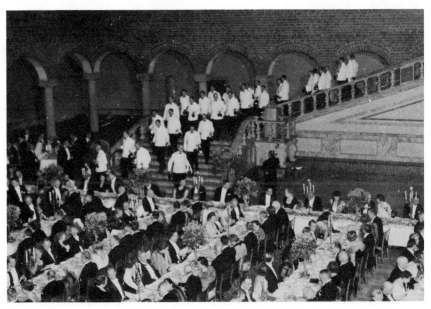

The banquet at the Stockholm City Hall, with waiters descending the marble staircase. At right on the landing is the rostrum from which each recipient gave an acceptance speech (Copyright Reportagebild)

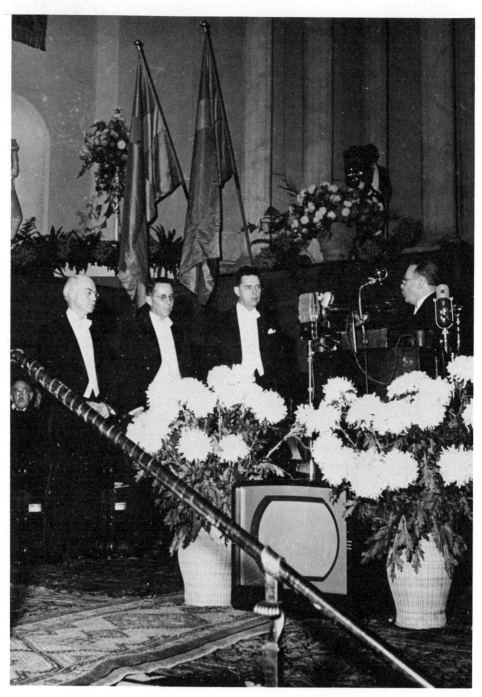

The laureates in Physiology and Medicine: (left to right) Kendall, Reichstein, Hench; at the microphone Professor Göran Liljestrand, sponsor for Physiology and Medicine (Copyright Reportagebild)

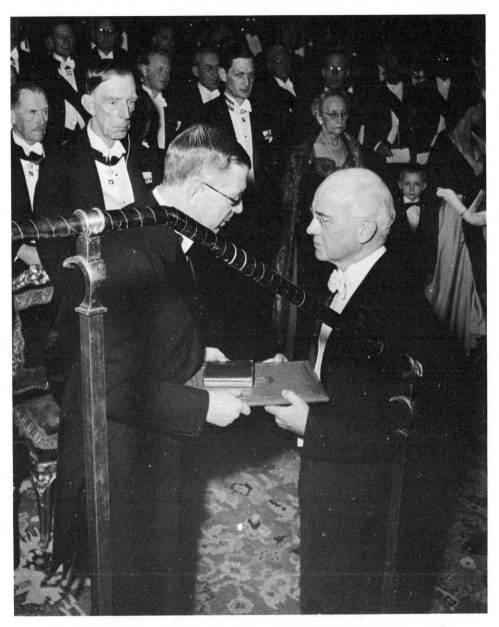

The Nobel Prize and citation presented by King Gustave VI (Copyright Reportagebild)

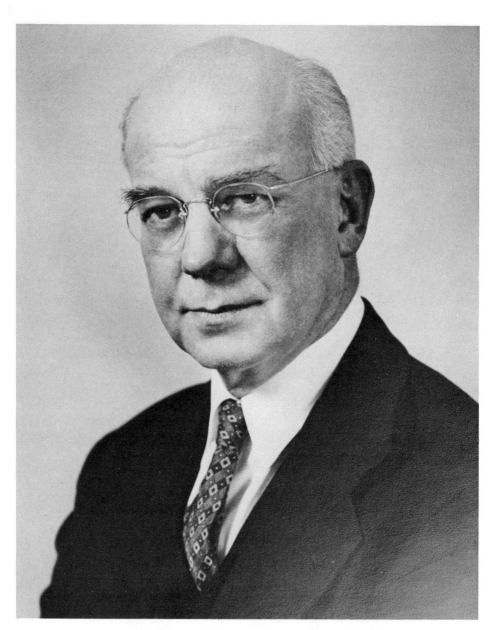

Edward C. Kendall (about 1949)

Nine

Some Effects of Cortical Hormones

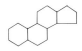

AGAIN WE WERE faced with a decision. Our staff and facilities were too small to permit an investigation of both hormones; which one should we choose? For therapeutic purposes desoxycorticosterone appeared to be the full equivalent of the amorphous fraction, and the synthetic compound was available in any required amount. The only source of the other hormone was the adrenal cortex. So long as this was so, the steroids with oxygen at carbon 11 would remain expensive and scarce. A bountiful supply of compounds A, B, E, and F was desirable for two reasons: first, very little was known about the physiologic activity of these hormones, and second, they were needed in the treatment of Addison's disease.

The decision was reached gradually. We had prepared several grams of each of the compounds and had learned much about their chemical and physical properties. They had lost much of the mystical, fanciful character that for so long had attended "the hormone" of the adrenal cortex. Dr. George Crile had lectured and written extensively about the "drive" that was imparted to the living organism by the adrenal gland. We held in our hand the hormone that initiated the drive and saw only a beautiful crystal.

The point is, we were dealing with a single chemical compound of known structure. There was no apparent reason why it could not be prepared from sources other than the adrenal cortex. Moreover,

Harold Mason, Willard Hoehn, Frank Stodola, Bernard McKenzie, and I had already done some work with steroids. We had prepared steroid derivatives from one of the bile acids and from cholesterol. The knowledge was a byproduct of the previous ten years' work, and it had value.

Finally, the aspect of the hormones of the adrenal cortex that was of greatest interest to the Mayo Clinic was their clinical application. This phase of the project could not be approached unless the hormones with oxygen at carbon 11 were available at a moderate cost. The decision was reached; we looked forward eagerly to the preparation of compounds A, B, E, and F from sources that were abundant and cheap. To achieve this new objective required almost ten years more, and before the work is described some other results should be recorded, lest they lose their place in the advance of time.

Viewed in retrospect, the decision to follow the fortunes of compound E rather than of the amorphous fraction was from every viewpoint the best course. But after the eventful pursuit of compound E, the problem of the hormone in the amorphous fraction still remained. How pure was our most active preparation of the amorphous fraction?

The conclusion we reached, that the hormone in the amorphous fraction was a steroid, was confirmed in 1953.* In its physiologic effect it closely resembled desoxycorticosterone, but it was much more active. The ratio of activity was estimated at 30:1; for our most active material this ratio was 16:1. On this basis our preparation contained about 50 percent of aldosterone, the name given the hormone. We prepared more than 1 gram of the compound in this state of purity.

The ideal arrangement for research in chemistry is to start a project with a group of workers who are able and willing to cooperate. As the investigation progresses, a jargon peculiar to the laboratory and to the problem is developed. Some of the properties of each new substance involved are: the melting point, specific rotation, spectrogram in the ultraviolet region, infrared spectrogram, molecular weight, and titration equivalent. These things are the subject matter of everyday conversation, most of which is mean-

---

* S. A. Simpson, J. F. Tait, A. Wettstein, R. Neher, J. von Euw, and T. Reichstein, *Experientia* IX: 333 (1953).

ingless to an outsider. For the group, however, the special vocabulary provides a shorthand that expedites the work. For example, one may refer to acid IA, or ketone 4.

If any member of the group has to be replaced, time is lost until the new member has acquired the special knowledge and can use the shorthand communication. Eight years after the beginning of the quest for cortin, Harold Mason transferred his attention from the adrenal cortex to assisting Dr. Russell M. Wilder with an investigation of the clinical aspects of a deficiency of thiamine.

We missed the steady hand and cool, conservative thinking of Harold Mason, but the direction of the work soon changed. There were new problems. Dr. Frank Stodola was appointed in his stead. Frank had received the degree of doctor of philosophy at the University of Minnesota and had carried on research for a year in the laboratory of Professor Butanant in Germany. He was familiar with the field of steroids, and he contributed three papers during the year he was in our laboratory.

Earlier I pointed out that, twenty years after the event, it matters not which details of the work came from our laboratory. However, the contribution of the dedicated laboratory workers deserves recognition. Of Dwight Ingle, the annual report for 1938, the year in which he left our laboratory, said: ". . . throughout the time during which Mr. Ingle has been associated with the work he has proved himself to be an able investigator whose work is thorough and reliable. He has shown the qualities of patience, persistence, resourcefulness and courage to a marked degree."

It is also recorded that "during 1937 Donald Krockow has conducted the physiologic assay of the solutions in a manner that has been beyond criticism. It is a job that requires his presence not only seven days a week including all holidays but he is obliged to make the trip to the Institute on several nights of almost every week. He has carried out the work faithfully and with excellent results."

In addition, Don conducted a long series of experiments that involved the influence of mineral salts on carbohydrate metabolism. This was an extension of the earlier work of Allers, Nilson, and Ingle. Drs. Mann, Bollman, and Flock were co-authors with me. The results demonstrated an intimate relationship between the metabolism of glucose and the distribution between tissue and fluids of potassium and phosphate ion. Cortical extract, insulin, and thyroxin modified this phenomenon. It was possible to express these effects in quantitative terms.

A measure of the quality of the service and devotion to duty of Don Krockow is given by the record of a dog that was adrenalectomized and pancreatectomized by Dr. Mann. Long and Lukens and other investigators had maintained such dogs for periods of a few weeks or months, but no longer. These dogs are hypersensitive to insulin, and they are especially susceptible to the development of sores and abscesses. Their appetite is capricious. They require constant observation and care. Don maintained our dog for three years. During this time many successive experiments were carried out to show the influence of compound E on the daily requirement of insulin, the effect of desoxycorticosterone and of compound E on carbohydrate metabolism and on mineral metabolism, and the influence of one on the other.

The dog was in excellent condition when Don was inducted into military service. After two weeks under the care of another technician the dog died.

Donald Krockow returned to the Mayo Clinic at the end of the war, but he could not resume his work. A neoplasm developed on his leg and metastasized rapidly; he died within a few months.

In 1938, in a paper published in *Endocrinology,* Dr. Conrad A. Loehner suggested that a deficiency of the adrenal secretion was involved in schizophrenia. Whether or not this was true, it suggested the possibility that some of our observations made concerning the effects of cortical hormones on the response of muscle to stimulation, carbohydrate metabolism, and the distribution of mineral ions might be carried over to biochemical processes in the nervous system.

In 1939 Dr. Ray Williams was added to the staff as a liaison member between the Rochester State Hospital in Rochester, Minnesota, and the Mayo Foundation. Most of his time was occupied with care of a group of patients under the observation of Dr. Wilder's group in a study of the clinical effects of a deficiency of thiamine, but Dr. Williams and I also carried out a study of the influence of the cortical hormones on a group of patients. The purpose of the work was to see whether there was a place in psychiatry for the use of these new agents. The results were not promising. We then turned to a more general investigation of the influence of mineral salts. A diet high in sodium content and low in potassium content was continued for ten days. This was then changed to the daily intake of salts high in potassium and low in sodium. Nothing of therapeutic value came out of the study, but several changes were of interest. All patients lost weight while they followed the high-potassium diet; all gained weight on the high-sodium diet.

The response to insulin that resulted in unconsciousness or convulsions was modified in a dramatic manner. When the intake of potassium was high, the response was greatly delayed or eliminated. When the intake of sodium was high, the time of response was shortened and the severity of the reaction markedly increased.

These effects were objective and were recorded on motion-picture film with a clock included to show the elapsed time. There were other subjective effects. The nurses on the ward could determine, simply by observation, which diet was being followed. When the intake of potassium was high, the patients were quieter, less troublesome, and much more subdued. When the intake of sodium was high, the reverse was true.

The reason for this type of study was to probe the scope of application of our new knowledge of the influence of mineral metabolism on physiologic processes. Many other attempts were made in this direction. Dr. Charles H. Slocumb employed the high-sodium, low-potassium diet for two patients who had rheumatoid arthritis in St. Mary's Hospital. Some abatement of the clinical symptoms was noted, but it was not striking. Moderate amounts of cortical extracts also were administered, but the effect did not warrant additional investigation.

In my contacts with the various sections of the Mayo Clinic, no opportunity was overlooked to find whether the cortical hormones could be of value in medicine. Dr. Robert D. Mussey's section was pleased with the use of the cortical extract in pernicious vomiting of pregnancy. Dr. Howard K. Gray credited the extract with saving the life of a patient in postoperative shock. But members of the section concerned with allergy and asthma found little use for the cortical hormones under the conditions that were employed.

Dr. Philip S. Hench, head of the department of arthritis at the Mayo Clinic, had many conferences with me. Each of us had a problem that was of top priority. His was to identify "substance X," which he was convinced could reverse the usual pattern of progress of the disease rheumatoid arthritis. Mine was to establish the value of the cortical hormones in clinical medicine.

In 1929 Dr. Hench had observed that patients who had rheumatoid arthritis sometimes were relieved of their symptons if jaundice developed. A few years later he noted that women with rheumatoid arthritis were frequently relieved if they became pregnant. A relationship between rheumatoid arthritis and pregnancy had been recognized by a few other clinicians, but whether the disease started from the time of pregnancy or was made better or worse by pregnancy was a matter of dispute.

Dr. Hench became convinced that the observations were of fundamental importance. He could not identify the agent responsible for relief of the symptoms of arthritis, and he was not certain whether the symptoms were caused by an excess of some substance or by a deficiency. He wondered whether a ductless gland was involved. He formulated a hypothesis and began a search for the unknown substance X.

In the summer of 1938 Dr. David Klein of the Wilson Laboratories, on one of his infrequent visits to Rochester, told me of some new work that had been carried out by Dr. Harry Edward Thompson and Dr. Bernard L. Wyatt at Tucson, Arizona. This was an attempt to devise a treatment of rheumatoid arthritis based on Hench's thesis of its relationship to jaundice. Hench had reasoned that, since idiopathic jaundice relieves rheumatoid arthritis, induced jaundice might produce the same effect. He had tried to induce jaundice in patients but had not succeeded. Thompson and Wyatt believed that the administration of bilirubin might be one way to reach the desired end, and they had approached Dr. Klein for a supply of that bile pigment. Dr. Klein had come to Rochester to inquire about the determination of bilirubin in blood and whether a solvent for bilirubin was known that would be satisfactory for injection into patients. I knew less about bilirubin than Dr. Klein did, and certainly no one in the Section of Biochemistry was simply sitting around waiting for the chance to do work on this subject.

90

On previous occasions when Dr. Hench and I had discussed the effect of jaundice on rheumatoid arthritis, I could not be of much assistance. But now he was asking for something tangible. He wanted to try the effect of induced jaundice on patients in Rochester and he needed help with the chemical aspects of the project: someone to prepare the solutions for injection in the blood.

Whether Dr. Hench's power of persuasion or intuition on my part was responsible, I became interested. Dr. Hench and Bernard McKenzie went to Tucson to see for themselves what the Wyatt Clinic had accomplished there.

Some work on bilirubin was then carried out in our laboratory. Though it did not prove effective, the important thing is that Dr. Hench had found someone in the Mayo Foundation who was interested in arthritis. He had tried to enlist the help of many others, but none had been able to devise an experimental approach that would shed light on his clinical observations. I was not prepared to stop the investigation of the adrenal cortex in favor of a study of rheumatoid arthritis. Nevertheless, it seemed possible that the explanation of Dr. Hench's observations might fall within the province of biochemistry, and that interested me very much.

In 1942 another method of producing jaundice came to Dr. Hench's attention. This was by administering an organic compound, lactophenin. The toxic effect of lactophenin had been known for some time, but Dr. P. Hanssen was the first[*] to employ the material to induce jaundice in patients who had arthritis. Jaundice developed in only about three of ten patients, but those who did become jaundiced seemed to be relieved of their arthritic symptoms.

This observation appeared to provide a beginning for study of the influence of jaundice on arthritis, and Dr. Hench was anxious to obtain some lactophenin for use with his patients. Since the compound was not available commercially, I asked McKenzie to make a large batch of the compound. It was prepared, crystallized, and delivered to Dr. Hench.

In January 1941 Dr. Hench and I had had a conference about arthritis. At the time both the chemical and the physiologic work was concentrated on compound E. The physiologic effects were

[*] *Acta Medica Scandinavica* 109:494 (1942).

striking, and I was much encouraged. It should be remembered that Hench had spent many years in the close study of arthritis. He was not familiar with the details of the work in my laboratory and knew nothing about compound E. On the other hand, I had spent ten years in the investigation of the chemistry of the adrenal cortex and knew nothing about rheumatoid arthritis. The exchange of ideas at the conference was not preserved, but it was at that meeting that we decided to try the effect of compound E on patients who had rheumatoid arthritis. This decision was recorded in Dr. Hench's pocket notebook. Neither of us realized that almost eight years would elapse before that decision could be carried out.

Study of the physiologic activity of the cortical hormones requires constant observation of the experimental animals. After Donald Krockow left the Institute of Experimental Medicine for military service physiologic investigation at the Institute was terminated. Between 1938 and 1942, however, Dr. Benjamin B. Wells and Dr. Roger Reinecke each carried out experiments of first importance.

Dr. Wells had received his M.D. degree in 1935 from the Baylor University College of Medicine. He did not enjoy clinical medicine but was enthusiastic about research in biochemistry. By means of his investigations the words "qualitative" and "quantitative" were placed in the vocabulary of these memoirs. He extended Ingle's work on atrophy of the thymus and adrenal glands; determined the concentration of mineral constituents of the blood after administration of compounds A, B, E, desoxycorticosterone, and the amorphous fraction; and, finally, made a series of experiments on the influence of these compounds on phlorhizin diabetes that have proved to be of classic stature.

For example, removal of the adrenal gland prevents the usual outpouring of glucose and urea produced by phlorhizin in the normal animal. If compound E is given with phlorhizin, the excretion of glucose is much increased and yet is not restored to that of a normal animal. If desoxycorticosterone is given with phlorhizin, the glucose in the urine is much less than it is after the administration of compound E. When 1.0 milligram of each is given with phlorhizin to an adrenalectomized rat, the loss of glucose is restored to that of a normal animal. Here is evidence of integration and synergism of two cortical hormones in the field of organic metabolism.

A similar observation concerned thyroxin. After the administration of phlorhizin to adrenalectomized rats, neither compound E nor thyroxin alone could increase the rate of excretion of glucose to the rate of normal rats, but the two hormones together could do so.

Wells also showed that, although fasted adrenalectomized rats under the influence of phlorhizin cannot convert their own proteins into glucose and urea at a rapid rate, they can utilize exogenous protein for this purpose. The amount of glucose excreted was increased in proportion to the weight of protein given to the rats. The inability to increase the rate of conversion of protein into glucose in the absence of the cortical hormones that had an atom of oxygen at carbon 11 was the explanation of much that had been observed previously. As mentioned, S. W. Britton had championed the hypothesis that the most important function of cortin was concerned with the metabolism of carbohydrates. This could not be proved to the satisfaction of all investigators, but by using the individual crystalline hormones, Wells was able to state in concise terms just what enzymes were influenced by these compounds.

Wells's work was carried out just when the hormones were available in generous amounts and when our thoughts about the activity of these compounds had reached maturity. In 1941 the University of Minnesota awarded him a Ph.D. degree.

Dr. Reinecke came to our laboratory after he had received the degree of doctor of philosophy from the University of Minnesota. He, like Dr. Wells, was interested more in research in biochemistry than in clinical medicine. His postgraduate work, which had to do with gluconeogenesis, provided a firm foundation for a study of the influence of the cortical hormones on carbohydrate metabolism.

Twelve years had passed since the preparation of the first potent extracts of the adrenal cortex, but standardization of such extracts was still in a state of confusion. Desoxycorticosterone provided a standard of comparison for the influence of such extracts on mineral metabolism, but that was only half the story. It had been found that there are many criteria for the influence of the hormones A, B, E, and F on carbohydrate metabolism, but all of them had a close relationship with the rate of deposition of glycogen in the liver of fasted adrenalectomized rats. We decided to explore this relationship.

Britton and H. Silvette, and also Long and his associates, had done much work on the influence of extracts of the adrenal cortex on the deposition of glycogen in the liver, but no method of bio-assay based on these results had been reported in the literature. As a result of the unremitting efforts of Reinecke such a method was devised.

Among the many sources of satisfaction provided by creative work in chemistry, two are particularly associated with the type of work carried out in our laboratory. One of these is isolating and making available some substance hitherto unknown, which is of importance in biology. Such a compound becomes incorporated in the thought and daily life of all future generations. The other is contributing a method of analysis or bio-assay. The field of useful-ness in the latter case is much more limited, but the sum total of the results that accrue from the use of such a method may be far-reaching.

The method devised by Reinecke has been adopted by all in-vestigators in the field. With slight modification, it is today the only bio-assay for the cortical hormones that influence carbohydrate metabolism. Reinecke and I published two papers. The first described the method for bio-assay; the second compared the activity of five steroids of the adrenal cortex. In view of what was to follow, it is interesting to note that there was less than a onefold difference between the activity of compounds A, B, and E.

Dr. Reinecke left the Mayo Foundation in 1942 to enter military service. After the war he accepted a position in the Medical School of the University of Puerto Rico, at Rio Piedras, Puerto Rico, where, as professor of physiology, he has continued his early interest in research and teaching.

Although experimental work on animals at the Institute of Experimental Medicine ended in 1942, a study of the effect of compound E on malignant tumors of the lymphatic glands was carried out in the laboratory of Dr. Fordyce H. Heilman, head of the Section of Bacteriology. The work was done in 1942, but the results were not published until 1944.*

* E. C. Kendall and F. H. Heilman, *Endocrinology* 34:416-420 (June 1944).

This project was started without fanfare and more as a matter of curiosity than as a serious attempt to cope with a tumor of high malignancy. In the course of routine examination of mice, Dr. Heilman found a large tumor that he believed was of lymphatic origin. He transplanted the tumor and then discovered that the percentage of successful transplants was 100. All transplants grew rapidly and all mice with the tumor died within a few days. After consultation and consideration, Dr. Heilman asked me whether I would be interested in carrying out a joint study of the effect of compound E on the tumor. Without hesitation I agreed to his suggestion.

This was the beginning of an interlude of high drama and great expectations. Compound E had a specific effect. Every mouse responded promptly. The tumors disappeared within 48 hours. Moreover, histologic examination showed that all the cells of the tumor responded. The influence of compound E appeared to depend on stimulation of the rate of catabolism of proteins to a degree which resulted in death of the malignant cells.

Whether or not this was the correct interpretation, compound E retarded for a week or more freshly implanted tumors from developing to palpable size, and other tumors that equaled half the weight of the mouse melted away in less than 36 hours. In ten or twelve cases the tumor did not return and the mouse appeared to be normal, but compound E was not the cure for neoplasms. The great majority of mice remained free of the tumor for only 10 to 14 days. Then, even though compound E was given continuously, the tumor slowly returned and was refractory to the hormone.

A restrained, conservative paper was sent to the editor of *Endocrinology* with the request that publication be withheld until further notice. Two years later a paper by J. B. Murphy and E. Strum on the influence of the adrenal gland on the lymphoid system rendered publication necessary.

Appearance of the paper started an argument, and the situation arose that we had most dreaded. We held almost the world's supply of compound E. The total amount was too small to permit distribution of the hormone. Moreover, not one patient who had a lymphatic tumor could be treated.

This was in 1944. The demand for cortical extract had increased to the point at which the formerly almost worthless adrenal gland now sold for five times the price of filet mignon. In this situation no pharmaceutical manufacturing company could afford to separate the crystalline hormones. There was only one satisfactory answer for all concerned—an unlimited source of compound E. The arguments and in some cases the hard feelings had to wait until the hormone was commercially available.

In 1938, when desoxycorticosterone became available and its striking effect on patients with Addison's disease had been shown, the implication was that the richest plum had been plucked from the tree by Professor Reichstein. It was ironical that an investigation such as ours, which was carried out on a broad basis with limitless material, should be undermined by the availability of a new, relatively simple steroid. No one could have foreseen that desoxycorticosterone would exert a marked effect on mineral metabolism; there was no basis for such a prediction; and yet clinical observations carried convincing evidence. There was a certain amount of disappointment and gloom around our laboratory.

Inevitably questions were raised. I attended a meeting of the board of governors to discuss the situation, and Dr. Donald C. Balfour and I had several lengthy and serious conferences. All these terminated in much the same way. My position was that the place of the hormones of the adrenal cortex in clinical medicine was still unknown, and I was convinced that it would be an important one. No one could produce evidence that this conclusion was wrong.

It has been my observation that it is better to have outsiders wave flags and do the shouting for some objective than for the research worker himself to do so. For the project under discussion, important support came from many clinical sections. Generous amounts of cortical extract had been furnished to them, and the results justified the confidence I expressed. Investigation of the cortical hormones was continued.

The interval during which desoxycorticosterone held top priority with research workers was of short duration. Failure of the compound to affect importantly any aspect of adrenal deficiency, other than mineral metabolism, served to emphasize the essential nature of the steroids that have an atom of oxygen at carbon 11. In short, the availability of desoxycorticosterone hastened the removal of this steroid from its high position and permitted those hormones with oxygen at carbon 11 to assume a place in the sun.

The meeting of the Federation of American Societies for Experimental Biology in 1941 was held in April at Chicago. I presented the latest results on the activity of compounds A, B, E, and F, expressed in qualitative and quantitative terms, and compared them with the results on the activity of desoxycorticosterone. The paper was well received. There was widespread interest in the new chapter that was beginning to unfold.

Ten

The Wartime Committee

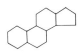

IN MAY 1941, a conference was held at Yale University at which the function of the adrenal cortex was discussed by representatives of almost all who had made contributions to this field. It was a serious and sober-minded group. The Second World War was well along in its second year, and we knew that the Medical Corps of both Army and Navy looked to this conference for guidance. At the conference it was stated on good authority that German scientists had beaten all others in the race to unravel the secret of the adrenal cortex. They were said to have made an extract that counteracted hypoxemia and permitted the pilots of the Luftwaffe to fly at 40,000 feet with impunity. Moreover, German submarines were then on their way to Buenos Aires to obtain bovine adrenal glands for preparation of the extract.

This information made us all feel like second-raters. If the chemists of the United States wanted to show what they could do, now was the time to start. It was later than we thought.

This hush-hush, secret, and most confidential report concerning scientists, airplane pilots, and submarines going out after adrenal glands was built up out of whispers and rumors that were completely without foundation. However, just enough evidence was placed before the conference to make these remarkable accomplishments seem plausible. In rats, an extract of the adrenal cortex did, in some degree, counteract hypoxemia. The extract also was reported to aid in treatment of shock and burns. Never before had the adrenal gland enjoyed such a monopoly of the spotlight. The hormones of the adrenal cortex furnished the beginnings of strength and the end of suffering.

During the summer, the war came closer, and first steps were taken to prepare for the entry of the United States if that event became unavoidable. The National Academy of Sciences appointed the National Research Council. Dr. A. N. Richards was made chairman of the committee in charge of medical research. Dr. Vannevar Bush headed the committee in charge of physics. Dr. William Mansfield Clark was chairman of the division of chemistry and chemical technology.

After these bodies had held several conferences with many groups of investigators, they chose three areas of investigation for top priority. These were, in order, compound E, penicillin, and anti-malarial agents. The good fairy had waved her wand; Cinderella was given the place of honor.

Progress in research is not produced by fanfare. The conversion of one complex molecule, such as a bile acid, into a still more complex substance, such as compound E, requires time, more time than anyone believed in 1941.

A meeting of chemists interested in the problem was held at Washington, D. C., on October 7, 1941, with Dr. Clark as chairman and about fifteen chemists attending. The purpose was to organize a group whose members would investigate the preparation of compound E, sharing their results in common. Some of those attending the meeting did not join but others did, and a committee was formed under the auspices of the National Research Council. Dr. William Mansfield Clark of Johns Hopkins University was chairman, and the other members were Drs. Hans T. Clarke, Columbia University; Everett Wallis, Princeton University; Caesar Scholz, Ciba; Louis Fieser, Harvard University; Karl Folkers, Merck and Co.; Randolph T. Major, Merck and Co.; Edwin Schwenk, Schering Corporation; R. D. H. Heard, McGill University; James B. Collip, Canadian National Research Council; Oskar Wintersteiner, E. R. Squibb and

Sons; Thomas F. Gallagher, University of Chicago; Werner Bergmann, Yale University; Edward C. Kendall, Mayo Foundation.

In 1941 not many laboratories in the United States were active in the field of research in steroids, but some members of the committee were outstanding teachers and research workers in universities and industries. I was happy at this turn of events. From the beginning of the investigation of the adrenal cortex I had looked forward to the time when we could work on the large-scale preparation of the hormones from sources other than the adrenal gland. Now that moment had arrived.

At the first meeting of the committee on the adrenal cortex it was decided that the first item on the agenda should be the preparation of compound A by "partial synthesis." Compound A was selected because its structure was less complicated than that of E. Any attempts to make compound A by "total synthesis" were to be postponed. (The terms "partial synthesis" and "total synthesis" are explained later.)

I returned to the laboratory after the conference, and within a few days McKenzie, McGuckin, and I completed the preparation of an intermediate compound on the long road from our starting material to compound A. We had begun this work three years earlier and had continued without interruption, but penetrating the boundary of the problem had consumed more time than we had anticipated.

A telephone call to Dr. Clark resulted in my return to Washington on October 26. Dr. Clark and Dr. Richards were much interested in my report. They believed that no time should be lost and decided to ask advice from Dr. Bush. Inquiry revealed that Dr. Bush was in New York and it was arranged by telephone that Dr. Richards, Dr. Clark, and I would meet with him that afternoon in the office of Dr. Frank B. Jewett, vice president of the American Telephone and Telegraph Company.

It was late afternoon before an airplane could take us to New York, and not until after working hours that we saw Dr. Bush and Dr. Jewett. They advised us to do three things: take out a patent to cover the new work; assign the patent to the Research Corporation of New York City; and ask Merck and Co. to prepare the compound under license from the Research Corporation. They too believed that no time should be lost. Another telephone call on that eventful day arranged a meeting with Howard Poillon, president of the Research Corporation, for eight o'clock that evening.

Mr. Poillon said that the Research Corporation would accept the patent when granted and agreed that Merck and Co. would be the most satisfactory pharmaceutical manufacturing company for preparation of the new compound. The next morning I met George W. Merck, president of the company. He was pleased with what had been done and arranged for me to see Dr. Randolph Major, the company's director of research, on October 29 in Chicago. Dr. Major welcomed the opportunity to have Merck and Co. undertake work in the field of steroids and promised to send one of their chemists to our laboratory.

The Merck chemist, Dr. Jacob van de Kamp, came to Rochester on November 1 and learned the details of the preparation of the first intermediate compound made from desoxycholic acid. This was the substance, first made by McKenzie, McGuckin, and myself, which permitted use of a bile acid as starting material for compound A. Merck and Co. prepared several kilograms of this compound, thus saving much time and labor in our laboratory.

The three years that followed were difficult. There was pressure from the desire to maintain our position of leadership in the committee under the National Research Council. There was loss of efficiency because well-trained men were taken from our laboratory and put into uniform by the military services. There were anxious moments caused by the passage of time. The adrenal cortex had been given first priority, but before long penicillin was available in ever-increasing quantities and atabrine was being used as a satisfactory antimalarial agent. Perhaps the greatest damage to the prestige of the committee, however, came in the fall of 1943, when the representative of Ciba Pharmaceutical Products on the committee reported that compound A had been prepared by Professor Reichstein.

That was a blow from which no recovery could be expected. Up to that time all members of the committee had concentrated their work on one phase of the preparation of compound A: to place an atom of oxygen on carbon 11. Many different avenues of approach had been tried, but no one had succeeded. We had reached that point at which it seemed that the whole problem would be solved if only we could surmount that major obstacle to the progress of the work.

Since Professor Reichstein had achieved the preparation of compound A, no one doubted that he would rapidly complete the last problem of the project: preparation of compound E. What had started out with high hopes and eager expectations now rapidly lost the quality of urgency. There was no doubt that the adrenal hormones had a place in medicine, but the United States was at war and the National Research Council was interested in medical problems that were important to prosecution of the war. It was necessary to face the facts: it was improbable that compound E could be made available for use during the remainder of the war. In June 1944 the last meeting of the committee was held in New York.

The reason for organizing the committee had not been to prove that compound E could be made; the purpose was to make it available for use in the Medical Corps of the Army and Navy. It was bad news, not only for the committee but also for the National Research Council, when the details of Professor Reichstein's method became known. The yield of compound A was 0.04 percent of the weight theoretically possible. That meant that the compound would be prohibitively expensive and available only in very small amounts.

Professor Reichstein had proved that compound A could be made, and this contribution had several important aspects. Among organic chemists it added still more prestige to a reputation already well established; it proved that the structure that had been assigned to compound A was correct; and it removed from the minds of the members of the committee a roadblock on the hormones of the adrenal cortex, for it showed that carbon 11 of the steroid nucleus could hold an atom of oxygen.

Nevertheless, even if Reichstein's method of preparing compound A could be much improved, the committee's objective of devising a method for the preparation of compound E in commercial quantities could not be met in time.

There is no question that the decision to form the committee in 1941 and the attempt to make compound E were correct. There is also no difference of opinion about the decision to dissolve the committee in 1944, but since compound E had not been prepared, there were a few whispers and some eyebrows were raised. The statement was circulated, though as far as I know not published, that the committee on the adrenal cortex was the only committee under the National Research Council that had failed to produce anything of value. When this statement was made it was apparently true, but time has shown that the judgment was superficial and premature.

Someone has made the remark that "no committee ever has written a great symphony." Creative chemistry can come to fruition only through the efforts of individuals, and in the search for knowledge time is of no importance. Although it was not recognized in 1943, an essential reaction that eventually made possible the large-scale production of compound E had been discovered in our laboratory.

In 1941 our laboratory was almost the only place in which compounds A, B, E, and F were available. Shortly after the committee was formed, the National Research Council asked me for one gram of pure crystalline compound E, to be sent, posthaste, to the corresponding committee in Great Britain for experimental purposes. When members of the National Research Council were asked what they expected the British to do with compound E, they were not clear; nevertheless they wanted it. The gram of compound E was given to the National Research Council and sent immediately to London. The British Medical Research Council presented it to Sir Henry Dale. There it rested. This is no reflection on the ability of British scientists. If the British Council had sent one gram of compound E to American scientists, it also would have rested unused.

An early action of the committee concerned standardization. This was prudent, since any synthetic material would have to be compared with the natural hormone. Dr. Sidney A. Thayer, a member of Professor Edward A. Doisy's laboratory in St. Louis University, was selected to carry out this work. Dr. Thayer came to Rochester and visited our laboratory. He chose the method developed by Reinecke and myself, and after the introduction of some minor changes he compared the activity of several samples of extracts of the adrenal cortex. These were furnished by the various companies or laboratories in which they were prepared. The result was a vindication of what I had believed but had never before been able to establish. I had sent two samples, one of bovine, and the other of porcine origin. Each was stronger than any of the extracts prepared in other laboratories.

If anyone had asked me whether the committee under the National Research Council was worth while, I would have answered an unqualified yes. The members, some of them old friends, came from widely separated institutions and were representative of organic chemistry in the United States and Canada. The feeling was engendered that if anything important happened, some member of the committee would know about it and report the matter at the next conference. This was a strong counteractant to rumors and hearsay. At each conference each member gave a summary of progress in his laboratory, and this also served to remove speculation and uncertainty. Finally, the formal presentation of reports and the informal conversation and questions were often of great help.

After June 1944 all members of the committee except Merck and Co. and the Mayo Foundation stopped work on the preparation of compound A. Among the pharmaceutical firms that had been members, Merck and Co. was the only one that retained an interest in the completion of the project. They had not accepted financial assistance from the National Research Council and they decided to continue the work on the same basis.

The motives that prompted me to undertake a study of the adrenal cortex in no way had decreased; rather, they had grown stronger. The board of governors of the Mayo Clinic still had faith in the project; much would be lost if the work was abandoned. The real problem, to determine the place of the hormones of the adrenal cortex in clinical medicine, still remained unsolved.

Eleven

Compounds A and E

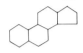

AT ONE OF the meetings of the committee on compound E, Dr. Randolph Major asked an innocent-sounding but really a leading question. It was "Why not have some member of the committee prepare a sample of compound A by whatever possible method?"

Up to that time each member had been preoccupied with a study of how to make compound A but had not taken time actually to make a sample of reasonable size. No one volunteered and in the end Merck and Co. undertook this project. Reichstein's method was known, and shortly before Dr. Major asked his question I had reported the new method devised in our laboratory. After consultation with members of the committee, Merck and Co. decided to make 5 grams of compound A by our method.

Mason and Hoehn, as already recorded, had converted one of the bile acids, desoxycholic acid, into a product that we hoped would be identical with a substance that had been obtained by degradation of compound A. This project was a substantial venture into the field of steroids, and we were encouraged when we found that we could improve on the work that was published in the literature. For example, one method for esterification of desoxycholic acid required this compound to be treated with 7.5 percent sulfuric acid in boiling alcohol for 16 to 18 hours. We found that this reaction was complete when the acid was treated in alcohol with dilute mineral acid

(0.10 N) at room temperature for only 2 hours. The difference in the two treatments was of more than academic interest. The ester made by boiling was of inferior quality and impurities were formed by the treatment itself. This was not an isolated instance. In fact, the field of steroids was an almost unexplored corner of organic chemistry.

It is now necessary to explain some chemical terms already used. These are "synthesis," "partial synthesis," and "total synthesis."

The word "synthesis" is not ambiguous. It means the preparation of a compound by man in the laboratory, as opposed to the formation of the same compound by natural processes. Examples are the making of acetic acid from ethanol or benzoic acid from toluene. Ethanol and toluene can both be built up from simpler compounds or even from the elements carbon, hydrogen, and oxygen.

The term "partial synthesis" may not be so clear. It does not mean that a product made by partial synthesis is only partially synthesized; in other words, that it is incomplete. It means that the compound is prepared by synthetic methods, but that the starting material is a natural product. Thus, heroin is made by alteration of morphine. This is a partial synthesis, with morphine as the starting material. The sex hormone testosterone can be prepared by alteration of cholesterol. Theoretically, the hormones of the adrenal cortex could be made by alteration—that is, by partial synthesis—from the bile acids as starting material.

But, the question may be asked, so long as the end product is made by synthetic methods, why is it necessary to add the word "partial"? The answer is that the advance in knowledge in organic chemistry and the genius of certain chemists have made it possible to elaborate heroin, compound E, strychnine, and many more very complicated compounds by "total synthesis," starting with simple compounds in the laboratory, which were not made by natural processes. The four compounds mentioned have all been made by total synthesis since 1951.

Preparation of a substance such as compound E by total synthesis, although possible, will be more expensive than preparation by means of partial synthesis, unless satisfactory natural starting material is not adequate. This now appears to be improbable. Bile from cattle, and certain tuberous roots, have been in supply sufficient to meet all requirements and this relationship can be maintained.

Another reason for preferring partial synthesis to total synthesis in the case of compound E was the time required. The problems involved in total synthesis appeared much more formidable than those concerned with partial synthesis. This assumption proved correct; after compound E had been made by partial synthesis, several years were required to devise the sequence of steps for total synthesis.

Three years before the committee under the National Research Council was formed, I had chosen one of the bile acids as starting material. With this precursor, the first problem was to change the position of an atom of oxygen from carbon 12 to carbon 11. Our plan of procedure was to remove the oxygen from its original attachment in such a way that one atom of bromine could be added to both carbon 11 and carbon 12. The two atoms of bromine were then replaced by one atom of oxygen, thus creating a new compound that was not the starting material. This was the product that caused my trip to Washington on October 27 and the arrangements with Merck and Co. and the Research Corporation that have been described.

Curiously enough, the direction of events that led to a method for the preparation of compound A on a commercial basis was determined by the fact that bromine was added to the bile acid after removal of the oxygen from carbon 12.

When Professor Reichstein's method for the preparation of compound A was revealed to the committee in 1943, I was most interested to learn that his starting material was the same bile acid we had used. He removed the atom of oxygen at carbon 12 by a procedure almost identical with ours and prepared exactly the same intermediate compound to which we had added bromine. Instead of adding bromine, however, he added hypobromous acid. This resulted in the addition of oxygen to carbon 11 and of bromine to carbon 12. Subsequent removal of the bromine created the product with oxygen at carbon 11. It was all straightforward and unambiguous. The only undesirable aspect of the method was the low yield of the compound. Had we used Professor Reichstein's sequence of steps we too could have prepared compound A, but our yield would have discouraged further investigation. Fortunately we added bromine and thereby made the first of a large number of steroid derivatives—the 3, 9-epoxy series—that culminated in a commercial method for the preparation of compounds A and E.

With the help of Dr. Jacob van de Kamp from Merck and Co., the grants from the Research Corporation, and the approval and support of the Mayo Clinic, we continued our study of steroids derived from bile acids. But for us there was no short cut, no clear result, and no course that could be charted and followed.

The pronoun "we" has been frequently used in this account because the work was carried on by a group. It is almost impossible for one person to maintain such an investigation. The work is subdivided, and it changes as progress is made. Let us assume that a compound, made in step 14 of the partial synthesis, occupies the most advanced position on June 1. This may be superseded by step 15 on June 30, but it is more probable that step 15 will not be discovered before October 1 or perhaps December 31. In the meantime, someone must carry out preparations of steps 1 to 14 and have material in quantity so that step 15 may afford intermediate compound 16. Steps 1 to 14 can be carried out by any competent chemist. The instructions are available. On the other hand, only a creative genius can advance step 14 to step 15. The project becomes a problem in organization. When the team has been developed, progress is limited only by the creative ability of its members.

In January 1942, the Research Corporation made Dr. Lewis Libman Engel available as a member of our laboratory group. This was an addition to our personnel, but, as the war effort expanded, more and more pressure was placed on all who could contribute. Bernard McKenzie volunteered and was accepted by the recruitment branch of the Army. That was a dark and cheerless day in my life, but the work was progressing and I could not abandon the project. Dr. Vernon R. Mattox came to the laboratory in July to replace McKenzie. Then, for some reason, still unknown, the Army revised its decision in regard to McKenzie. Nevertheless, Dr. Mattox stayed on. The members of the group then were Engel, Mattox, McKenzie, McGuckin, and myself.

The staff was twice augmented temporarily in 1942. Early in

110

the year Lewis Hastings Sarett spent three months with us. He had joined Merck's staff of research chemists after receiving his Ph.D. from Princeton University. In June, Richard Baldwin Turner, who had just received the same degree from Harvard University, joined us.

Dr. Sarett succeeded in identifying the chemical structure of the new compound made by replacement of two atoms of bromine with one atom of oxygen. This structure had remained uncertain for some months, and to have the nature of that particular intermediate compound established without question was important, since it was a labile substance. Dr. Turner was responsible principally for the proof of the structure of a close relative to the new compound, which McKenzie and I shortly afterward converted into still another steroid derivative. The whole group was puzzled over the chemical structure of this one for several months. It gives me great satisfaction to be able to say that, by good fortune, it was I who suggested the correct chemical structure for this compound, which proved in the end to hold the key to the addition of oxygen to carbon 11 with a high yield of the compound. (Just for the sake of the record, it was Δ11–3,9 epoxycholenic acid.)

To make this compound from our starting material required many steps and the yield was not satisfactory. We wanted to use the same starting material but to arrive at the compound by steps that gave higher yields. The answer to this problem came from a meeting of the committee on compound E. By chance, Dr. Wintersteiner mentioned that Dr. Schwenk had used selenium dioxide as an oxidizing agent. At the next meeting of the committee Dr. Schwenk furnished the details. There was no apparent application of Dr. Schwenk's work to the partial synthesis of compound A, but on the train that night it occurred to me that this might provide a new approach to our problem. It was soon evident that with selenium dioxide we could sidestep the undesirable intermediate compounds and prepare the Δ11 cholenic acid with an excellent yield. This is one example of the help derived from the committee that was mentioned in the preceding chapter.

Dr. Mattox, Dr. Engel, and I went a step farther by adding bromine to the new derivative of cholenic acid at carbon atoms 11 and 12. This time the bromine on carbon 11 could be replaced

111

selectively with oxygen. As a last alteration, McGuckin and I re-established the original steroid structure, but with oxygen on carbon 11. This was achieved during the last weeks of 1943.

There were many frustrating days while other changes in the partial synthesis were devised, but in February 1944 McGuckin made a small amount of compound A. During that same month he was inducted into the Navy. He was sorely missed. Although he had to his credit only two years of junior college work, Warren McGuckin was one of the most efficient workers in the laboratory. He had a "chemical nose" and could smell out the pathway through a tangle of obstructions. He was courteous and cooperative under all circumstances, completely reliable and efficient, oblivious of the clock on week days, Sundays, and holidays. His place in our laboratory remained unfilled for many years.

On a cold, frosty morning early in 1944, I met the train that brought Dr. Randolph Major to Rochester. He came to discuss the preparation of compound A by our new method. This attempt to manufacture the hormone was to be on a large laboratory scale. Jacob van de Kamp and S. M. Miller of Merck and Co. were assigned to this work with the expectation that from the starting material they would be able to make at least 5 grams of compound A.

The prospects that lay before them were not pleasant. In the first place, if they encountered trouble and could not obtain our yield of each intermediate compound, they would be blamed. In the second place, they were to be occupied with this assignment for a year or more and thus isolated from the chance to work on other problems that seemed more worthwhile and rewarding. But they could protect themselves in one way. They could start with such a large amount of bile acid that they could not fail to finish with 5 grams of compound A. This they did.

If there is another pair of chemists more friendly and efficient than "Jaap and Monty," I do not know where to find them. I know from experience that they talk freely to each other, but not one word about what they are doing reaches any unauthorized ear.

They were furnished full directions and proceeded from one step to the next without exchanging a word with me until late summertime. I visited their laboratory, went over their experiences, explained how to separate two compounds through the difference in the rate of crystallization, and left them to finish.

In our laboratory during 1945, several new reactions were studied, the method of preparation of compound A was much improved, and we looked forward to the time when it would be available for physiologic and clinical investigation.

Once again our group felt the pressure of the war, when the National Research Council transferred Dr. Turner to work in Boston on the preparation of antimalarial agents. This transfer of personnel to work regarded as more important for prosecution of the war was in keeping with the dismissal of the committee on the adrenal gland. But to us it was another reminder that the spotlight had moved on. In August 1945, Dr. Gerard A. Fleisher came to our laboratory to replace Dr. Turner.

In December 1945 I visited Merck and Co. for a conference with Dr. Major. More than a year and a half had passed since van de Kamp and Miller had started to make compound A and they were ready to report. They had followed our directions and had matched our yields of the many intermediate compounds. The final yield of compound A, however, was not about 5 grams; it was 97.3 grams. The increase resulted from improvements in the efficiency of several of the steps involved. The final yield was 0.376 percent.

There were congratulations and broad smiles. Compound A was the most complicated molecule, requiring more steps than any other compound made by a pharmaceutical company. Its manufacture on a large scale was taken as assurance that preparation of compound E soon would be possible. Interest in the hormones of the adrenal cortex rose rapidly, and plans were made for an announcement to the world of science.

The annual meeting of the Federation of American Societies for Experimental Biology was to be held at Atlantic City in March 1946. Dr. Major and I made arrangements with the program committee for a session on compound A on the day preceding the annual meeting, and the announcement of the session, with Dr. Cyril Norman Hugh Long as chairman, appeared in the agenda. Little more than two months remained before the meeting, but we hoped that some physiologic or clinical results could be presented.

Compound A has a definite chemical structure that is always the same whether it is made in the adrenal gland of an animal or prepared by partial synthesis from bovine bile. Ingle had shown that A maintains the ability of muscle to perform work; Long and his associates had first demonstrated the influence of A on carbohydrate metabolism; Ingle and Wells had found that A causes atrophy of the thymus and adrenal glands; and Reinecke had measured the ability of A to permit deposition of glycogen in the liver of adrenalectomized rats.

For these reasons it seemed probable that compound A would be of value in the treatment of adrenal deficiency. However, compound E was regarded as a big brother of A. This did not mean that E was ten or twenty times more effective than A. Many of those in a position to have an opinion thought that E might be two or perhaps three times as active as A. Stated in terms of daily dose, if 20 milligrams of E were required for substitution therapy, 40 or 60 milligrams of A should be equally satisfactory.

The meeting at which the work on compound A was presented was well attended. Professor Reichstein happened to be in the United States and was present. There could be little critical discussion about the chemical work; Merck and Co. had confirmed all our statements about the procedure and the yields. What was of interest to most of the audience, and particularly to Dr. Major and his associates at Merck, were the clinical results. All the preliminary results reported were in agreement with the conclusion of Dr. Edwin J. Kepler of the Mayo Clinic. He had found that in the treatment of Addison's disease compound A has no value. His pronouncement was made more significant and irrevocable by the fact that he had telephoned the Mayo Clinic within the hour. His results were based on the use of 200 milligrams of A for a daily dose. As we walked out of the auditorium Dr. Konrad Dobriner of the Sloan-Kettering Foundation remarked to me, "This meeting never should have been held. Now no pharmaceutical company can be persuaded to try to make compound E."

March 1946 was a low point in the development of compound E. The difference between the structures of compounds A and E consists of one atom of oxygen. To almost everyone it seemed improbable that this difference could be important enough to justify the attempt to make compound E. However, one example among the steroids of the adrenal cortex was encouraging. It was well established that the addition of one atom of oxygen completely changed the properties of desoxycorticosterone. The addition of oxygen to carbon 11 changed desoxycorticosterone into compound A. Who could say what would be the effect of the addition of oxygen to carbon 17 of compound A? This would convert A to E but would that be worthwhile?

There never was any question in my mind about continuing the project to make compound E. Our laboratory had separated more than 30 grams of compound E from the extracts of the adrenal gland. We had used it on animals and for chemical work and had given generous amounts to other investigators. Our results strongly indicated that there would be a place for it in clinical medicine.

The fear that no pharmaceutical company would attempt to make compound E was not substantiated. Dr. Major called a dinner meeting of members of Merck and Co. on October 24, 1946. Dr. C. N. H. Long and I were included, and all aspects of the situation were discussed. Some months earlier a decision to prepare 5 grams of compound E had been made. This decision was confirmed by all present. I remarked that I was in favor of the plan to make compound E, but that I was much concerned about what could be accomplished with 5 grams. It would not be wise to give the entire amount to one investigator. If 2.5 grams was given to each of two clinicians, that quantity would be too small to repeat an experiment, regardless of whether the result was positive or negative. Dr. Long agreed with me in this discussion, and it was decided to continue work on the preparation of the first steps. This material would be held until a satisfactory method had been devised to add an atom of oxygen to carbon 17 of the steroid nucleus.

Again the burden of this new venture was placed in the hands of van de Kamp and Miller. They were now experts in the field and were the best qualified to carry on the work. Whether it was in jest or not I was never certain, but they pretended to be much annoyed at this second term of banishment from current events and opportunities to work on something of value. They were now steroid chemists and nothing else.

The conversion of a bile acid into compound E is something

like the construction of a building. The foundation must be finished before the first floor can be started, and so with the second floor and all that follows. Discovery of a method for the addition of oxygen at carbon 11 provided our laboratory with a strong foundation, but five other alterations were necessary before compound E would be complete. During 1946 these were taken under study, and attempts were made to find the best procedure for each one. This type of research is time-consuming. Only by continued trial is it possible to establish the finer shades of response given by the intermediate compound under investigation. We did make progress, but the chemical facts that we sought were not to be found in any library; they could be obtained only through continued meticulous research in the laboratory.

When Dr. Sarett left Rochester in 1942 he returned to the research laboratory of Merck and Co. Each time I went there his laboratory was one of the first places I visited. Had anyone watched closely, he would have wondered why I was in such a hurry to see Sarett and probably concluded that something was happening that required immediate attention. So there was. Dr. Sarett was a good chess player. We both enjoyed correspondence chess and played many a game by mail. Whenever I was in Rahway I liked to drop in and tell him what my next move would be. He had a small set of chess men in his laboratory and we would take a few minutes to discuss the game.

However, no one could have accused either of us of retarding the advance of science by overindulgence in chess. The driving force that made the wheels go around for both of us emanated from the desire to finish project E. Work in the two laboratories was entirely independent, and the details were not discussed until after each step was completed.

While compound A still held top priority in our laboratory, Sarett attempted conversion of A to E through a series of steps that involved conversion of a hydroxyl group at carbon 20 to a ketone. He was successful and at the end of December 1944 he prepared the first few milligrams of compound E made from starting material not present in the adrenal cortex. However, the yield was much too small to provide a method for large-scale manufacture.

116

This was a duplication of the situation in 1943 when the committee on the adrenal cortex learned of the preparation of compound A by Professor Reichstein and his associates. Here was tangible evidence of the ability of this young chemist to bring a difficult project to a successful conclusion. If the prestige of Dr. Sarett were charted, one would see a curve rising rapidly with time. The first big dot to mark that curve would be the partial synthesis of compound E. His work confirmed the structure previously assigned to compound E. This removed all doubt. Carbon 17 could hold an atom of oxygen. We were working in the right direction. However, the original objective still remained. The yield obtained by Sarett's method was too small to permit the commercial production of compound E. For that, further research was necessary.

During the year 1947 Dr. Sarett devised a much improved method to place an atom of oxygen at carbon 17. The final stage of the preparation of compound E now was within sight.

One major obstacle remained. This was the introduction of a double bond in ring A of the hormone. Ten years previously we had shown that removal of the double bond in the hormones of the adrenal cortex destroyed the physiologic activity. Now we were faced with the problem of introducing that essential grouping, for it is not present in the bile acid that was our starting material. Dr. Mattox and I had studied this problem in 1945, and in the spring of 1947 this work came to fruition in a most satisfactory way.

In the preparation of compound E it was necessary to carry the starting material through 30 successive steps. There was some loss at each step, but let us say that we reached step 28 with 1000 grams of material. There was little loss at step 29; we still would have almost 1000 grams with which to work, but when we finished step 30 at least two-thirds of it would have been destroyed. If we could gather together 300 grams of compound E we would have to be satisfied. No sequence of steps was available that would give a satisfactory yield. The method now known as the Mattox-Kendall procedure afforded more than 900 grams of compound E from 1000 grams of intermediate step 28. This was the last necessary contribution for the partial synthesis of compound E on a commercial scale.

We discovered a new way to form a double bond. This method

could be used with many compounds other than E, and much time was spent in a detailed study to find the conditions required to give the maximal yield not only of E but of A and other steroids.

In the spring of 1948 Dr. van de Kamp brought to Rochester a sample of compound E that he had made on a small scale in Rahway. He was well pleased with the pure white crystals. His exuberant spirits no doubt resulted from the satisfaction that comes from completing a difficult task beset with pitfalls and problems.

For the initial large-scale application of this method, Merck and Co. sent Monty Miller to Rochester with the intermediate compound preceding the last step. This was converted into compound E in my laboratory, and Monty took the hormone back to Rahway when he returned. I remember this incident well: Monty and I worked all day on Thanksgiving Day, 1948.

Only those who have worked in a chemical laboratory similar to that of Merck and Co. can appreciate the contribution made by van de Kamp and Miller. For compound A the starting material, desoxycholic acid, weighed 65 pounds. There was not much change in weight in the first few steps, but after many months of work the entire product could be contained in one small flask. If the flask were broken at that stage and the material lost, the project would have to be started over from the beginning. To continue under this psychic strain for more than a year requires more than technical ability and more than unusual patience and persistence; it requires strength of character. Had these two men failed in their assignment it is questionable whether anyone else would have ventured to make the attempt. Dr. Dobriner's prediction might well have come true. It is probable that within a few more years compound E would have become available, but that would have changed the most important chapter of these memoirs.

In the partial synthesis of compound E the introduction of an atom of oxygen at carbon 17 required many more additional steps. For this reason the weight of the starting material was increased almost twenty times.

A new therapeutic agent does not happen suddenly. It may appear to reach the prescription department of retail drug stores as a brand-new product, and it may receive wide publicity within a matter of weeks or even of days, but the record will show that years of work were required before the retail druggist could receive the new product.

Dr. Major had suggested that compounds A and E be prepared. I do not know what obstacles were raised when compound A was found to be without value, but I do know that Dr. Major guided project E past all difficulties.

Merck and Co. lived up to the highest ideals of a manufacturing company when they persisted in the project to make compound E available on a scale sufficient to permit a study of its physiologic properties. Without assurance of financial return, their contribution was a venture into the unknown.

When the new laboratory of the Sloan-Kettering Institute was opened on April 16, 1948, I was in New York to attend the ceremony, and had a conference with Dr. Major. He said that a meeting to be held on April 29 would include a group of clinicians interested in the hormones of the adrenal cortex and he asked me to be present. I accepted his invitation.

Compound E had been made available. Now nothing blocked the way of a clinical study on an impressive scale. The day to which I had looked forward since 1938 had arrived. I entered that after-dinner conference with suppressed emotion and with hopeful expectation that this meeting would mark the end of the long road that we had traveled since 1930.

These expectations were not realized. As the evening progressed, the atmosphere seemed to turn from cool to frigid. The spirit of adventure was at no time manifest. Whether it was fear of the use of a compound that had cost so much to prepare, or hesitancy to be associated with a clinical investigation that probably would result in failure was not evident. Dr. Randall G. Sprague requested a small amount of compound E for use in a study of Addison's disease, but no one suggested that compound E be tried in any of the hundred-odd diseases for which cortisone is used today. Some members of the group said that they did not care to use compound E even for Addison's disease unless some derivative could be prepared that would make the hormone soluble in water.

No ray of light could pierce the gloom of that gathering. It re-

119

minded one of W. E. Henley's "Invictus": ". . . the night that covers me, Black as the Pit from pole to pole." April 29, 1948, was for me the low point of the entire investigation of the adrenal cortex.

It must also have been a time of trial for Dr. Major. Before the meeting he had warned me that unless some definite use for compound E could be found, he was not confident that Merck and Co. would continue this project. Dr. Major was not able to attend the conference, but any report that reached him must have been pessimistic.

It soon became evident that the opinions expressed at the meeting in New York were quite in keeping with the attitude of most clinicians. It seemed that Dr. Dobriner's remark at Atlantic City should be changed to: "No one will be interested in using compound E, even if it is available."

Whether the failure of compound A had produced this devastation among clinicians is a question, but certainly no one suggested an important use for compound E other than for Addison's disease from April 29 until September 21 of 1948.

Twelve

Arthritis

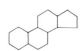

WHEN I RETURNED to Rochester, I soon shook off the pessimism created by the meeting. Several manuscripts, already late, had to be put into shape for publication and sent to journals. More study was given to attempts to increase the yield of compound E, and arrangements were made with Dr. Randall G. Sprague for the trial of compound E on a patient who had Addison's disease.

One day in August I met Dr. Hench in the lobby of the clinic building, and he asked, "How is compound E coming along?"

I replied, "Well, you may be surprised one of these days. Compound E is going to be available."

Shortly after this I took a few days off at our cottage at Lake Zumbro. On Thursday I went into the laboratory and found a note asking me to call Dr. Hench. Whether I tried to make the call then and could not reach him or whether I postponed making it I do not remember. What I do distinctly remember is the sense of urgency that came over me on my return to the cottage. After dinner I decided to call Dr. Hench that evening instead of waiting until I returned to Rochester on Monday.

The nearest telephone was in a farmhouse about two miles away. It was an old-fashioned wall telephone, the kind that was equipped with a crank to attract the attention of the operator. I still recall the discomfort of the following forty-five minutes. The mouthpiece was placed so that I had to stand all the time Dr. Hench and I were engaged in the discussion that we now know marked the real turning point in project E.

The conversation concerned a patient, Mrs. G., who had rheumatoid arthritis. She had been given lactophenin in an attempt to induce jaundice, but she had not responded to the treatment. This was a disappointment. The patient was discouraged, and morale in general sank. At this time another patient who had arthritis became jaundiced, and fortunately the jaundice brought about remission of the symptoms of arthritis. Mrs. G., much impressed by the obvious change for the better in the other patient, expressed the hope that something more could be done for her. Dr. Hench wanted to help Mrs. G., and when he recalled my remark that compound E would be available soon, he decided to administer the hormone to her, if this could be arranged.

The first use of compound E in a case of rheumatoid arthritis was the burden of our conversation. I was eager to cooperate in such a venture. However, it would be necessary to secure an adequate supply of the hormone. There was compound E in my laboratory, but it was not sufficient to permit prolonged treatment of even one patient. Dr. Hench needed an immediate answer. Should he tell Mrs. G. that nothing more could be done at this time, or could he tell her that if she would stay in Rochester a further attempt would be made to relieve the symptoms of arthritis? The conversation was concluded by my promise to provide sufficient compound E to treat one patient.

The telephone operator informed me that the charge for the call was $1.14. I reimbursed the farmer and returned to our cottage at the lake.

September 1948 was a busy time for Dr. Hench. He had been invited to give the annual oration before the Heberden Society of London and was occupied with duties concerned with that important occasion. However, nothing could take priority over the treatment of rheumatoid arthritis with compound E. In a conference held to decide some essential details, three important decisions were made. These were: first, to use free compound E rather than the 21-acetate ester; second, to inject, intramuscularly, the pulverized material suspended in isotonic solution of sodium chloride; and third, to administer 100 milligrams each day. At the time, we could not know how important each of these decisions was. Within a few months it became evident that we had chosen well.

Procurement of compound E was my responsibility, and at first several questions lacked satisfactory answers. The most important question concerned compound E itself. The hormone was potentially available from the laboratory of Merck and Co. but in September 1948 the amount that was ready for use was limited to a few grams. It did not occur to me that there would be any hesitancy on the part of Merck and Co. to use some of the hormone for an attempt to relieve the symptoms of rheumatoid arthritis. However, the company's medical department knew full well the value of each gram of compound E in terms of time, effort, and money. Everyone concerned was eager to find a use for the hormone, but a telephone call to Rahway revealed some skepticism about its value in rheumatoid arthritis. Dr. Major was not available, and in his absence the medical department requested a rationale from Dr. Hench for the use of compound E in rheumatoid arthritis.

This was a reasonable request, but at the time it was not possible to write a convincing answer. Sufficient compound E was available to start treatment of Mrs. G., but it was uncomfortably evident that unless there was a beneficial effect, it would be difficult to secure more of the hormone for treatment of rheumatoid arthritis. Still, it was also clear that if Dr. Hench's reply could be reinforced by a *fait accompli,* all would be well. Dr. Hench complied with the request for the rationale. After a short delay 5 grams of compound E was sent by Merck and Co. to the Mayo Clinic.

The second problem was preparation of the hormone in its "free" form; that is removal of the acetate ester and suspension of the compound in the form of a fine powder in isotonic solution of sodium chloride. Removal of an acetate group from a compound is a common procedure in a chemical laboratory, but when this is carried out on material that costs $200 a gram, that is unusual. For obvious reasons we wanted to devise the most efficient method for this step.

It is possible to remove the acetate group from the acetyl ester of compound E by treatment with a base, but our first attempts were not satisfactory, and Dr. Mattox devised a method that employed acid aqueous alcohol. The yield of "free" compound E was about 75 percent. This meant that from every 4 grams of compound E acetate only 3 grams of compound E would be available for injection, but we believed that the "free" compound should be employed until some other form of the hormone was shown to be equally effective.

Preparation of the first several grams of "free" compound E proceeded without difficulty, except for one aspect. At least 48 hours were needed for removal of the acetate group. Such a period required careful arrangement of a schedule, since we were resolved that no patient would be deprived of treatment, even for one day, because of lack of compound E.

It was not necessary to carry out an investigation of the last step. This was to grind compound E to a fine powder and suspend it in sterile isotonic solution of sodium chloride. This method was a practice of long standing and had been shown to be satisfactory. The concentration of compound E in suspension was 1 gram in 50 milliliters of isotonic solution of sodium chloride. This provided 100 milligrams of the hormone for each injection of 5 milliliters.

I asked Dr. Harold Mason to make up the suspension of the first gram of compound E, which he did. All the 150 grams subsequently used I prepared myself.

The suspension of the first gram of compound E was sent to St. Mary's Hospital on Friday, September 17, 1948. I was keenly aware that the day of reckoning had arrived. The question of whether compound E could influence the symptoms of rheumatoid arthritis was to be answered by Mrs. G. If a favorable effect could be demonstrated, the optimal dose readily could be determined. But if no influence on the disease could be shown under the conditions employed, then it was not probable that any other method of administration would give results that were more encouraging.

The clinical trial of compound E was similar to that of compound A, except in one respect. In the case of compound A it had been possible to justify failure of activity by the thought that, after all, this was only compound A and we could still look forward to the clinical trial of compound E. But in September 1948 we had in hand that elusive hormone, compound E. We had reached the end of the road. The answer had to be yes or no.

It was a comfort that the answer would be disclosed in a matter of days, but doubt and uncertainty would remain until those days had passed. I had a strong inclination to call St. Mary's Hospital each day but managed to refrain until the end of the week.

Imagination is a phenomenon that is the basis of creative genius. It is an essential ingredient of progress, and yet it can lead to the generation of hope and expectation that have no substance in fact. Experience can develop the power to control one's imagination, but it is difficult to contemplate in a detached and impersonal manner the approach of a moment that could determine the direction and pattern of the remaining days of one's scientific career.

After eighteen years of uninterrupted effort, such a time had arrived in my life. There were 3,000,000 patients in the United States who had rheumatoid arthritis. Was it possible that compound E could help control this destructive disease? These people were not united in an organization with representatives who could speak for them. Nevertheless, even though they were silent, they had an appeal as strong as if they had been united and vocal. I tried not to think of Mrs. G. as the appointed delegate of all who had rheumatoid arthritis. She was a single patient; it would not be wise to expand the answer she gave.

It seemed certain to me that if Mrs. G. responded favorably to compound E, that result would be apparent by Saturday, September 25. I called St. Mary's Hospital and talked to Dr. C. H. Slocumb, who was in charge of the hospital service of Dr. Hench's section of medicine. Mrs. G. had been given daily injections of a suspension of compound E. She had responded on the second day and had continued to improve as time passed. The answer to my inquiry was an unqualified yes.

"Initial doses of compound E were 100 mg. daily (50 mg. twice a day). On the morning of September 21, before the first injection . . . the patient could hardly get out of bed; once she tried to walk; it was too painful, and so she remained at rest. But on September 23, after two days of use of compound E, she woke with much less muscular stiffness and soreness, rolled over in bed easily for the first time in weeks and noted increased strength and appetite. Although she felt much better subjectively and the fibrositic component seemed to be much decreased, articular tenderness was unchanged. On the next day (September 24) improvement continued and we found her exercising, raising her hands over her head, previously im-

125

possible. She visited several patients to demonstrate her changed condition. Painful stiffness was gone. 'My muscles feel stronger, and my appetite is very good.' After six days she had lost almost all her stiffness; articular tenderness and pain on motion were markedly reduced. The next afternoon (September 28) she shopped for three hours downtown, feeling tired thereafter but not sore or stiff. She noted a sense of well-being: 'I have never felt better in my life.' "*

This result was only a beginning. But to an optimist it was significant. The coming months would confirm or deny this first indication, but now we had more than a rationale for the use of compound E in the treatment of rheumatoid arthritis.

It is difficult to describe the turmoil and emotion in the mind of Dr. Hench at that time. For many years he had believed that the symptoms of rheumatoid arthritis are reversible. For years he had predicted that an unknown agent, "substance X," could bring about such a reverse. Ever since January 1941 he had looked forward to the day when he could investigate the effect of compound E on the symptoms of rheumatoid arthritis. Was "substance X" a product of the adrenal gland? Was "substance X" compound E? The effect of the compound on the condition of Mrs. G. indicated that now we had an experimental tool that could be used to explore these questions.

I visited Mrs. G. at St. Mary's Hospital. When Dr. Hench introduced me, he remarked that I had carried out the chemical work on the new compound that had been given to her. She turned toward me and said, "Let me shake your hand."

I met Mrs. G. on September 27, and the very next day Dr. Hench had to leave Rochester for England. He did not return until December 23. The intervening months were filled with frequent communications between Dr. Hench and Dr. Slocumb, in the form of letters, cablegrams, and telephone calls, reflecting the progress of the clinical investigation. They recorded our hope and frustration, anticipation and postponement, failure and success. To Dr. Hench they must have seemed like a nightmare. But there was a happy ending and further details of a distressing experience are best omitted.

In New York City, just before embarking for England, Dr. Hench had a conference with Drs. James Carlisle and Augustus Gibson of

* *Archives of Internal Medicine,* 85:545-666 (1950).

Merck and Co. The results were an additional supply of compound E and a visit to St. Mary's Hospital by Dr. Carlisle. He came to Rochester to see for himself how patient number 2 would respond to treatment with compound E. Patient number 2 responded in a manner like that of Mrs. G. Dr. Carlisle was satisfied that compound E was effective. That good news was sent to Rahway without delay.

During October and November, 1948, treatment of patients 1 and 2 was continued, and patients 3 and 4 were added to the group. All of them had responded in a sequence that was now recognized as typical. These results raised three important questions. Does compound E have a specific and unequivocal effect on the symptoms of rheumatoid arthritis? Is there a place for compound E in the armamentarium of clinical medicine? What must be done to answer the two preceding questions?

These three questions were asked and answered in the executive office of Merck and Co., the Department of Research and Development of Merck and Co., my laboratory at the Mayo Foundation, the meeting room of the board of governors of the Mayo Clinic, and St. Mary's Hospital.

In September of 1948 the value of research in the field of steroids was a matter of controversy. From the viewpoint of the pharmaceutical manufacturing company, the sale of steroid products had not rewarded the effort and expenditures that had been made. The experience with the hormones of the adrenal cortex was especially disappointing. Ciba and Co. and Organon had placed desoxycorticosterone on the market, but the volume of sales was small. Merck and Co. had made compound A, but as a pharmaceutical product it was without value. Merck had also produced compound E, generous samples had been sent to each one of a group of able clinicians, but no one had suggested any clinical condition for which large amounts of the hormone would be required. There was an inclination to face the facts and admit that the future of compound E was dark.

Now word came from the Mayo Clinic that compound E exerted a beneficial effect on rheumatoid arthritis. Should this preliminary report be accepted at face value and further exploration made? I do not know what opinions were expressed or how vigorously they were advanced or attacked, but the final decision was to assist the Mayo Clinic with sufficient compound E to answer the first two questions.

The first request received from the Mayo Clinic for project "rheumatoid arthritis" was for 5 grams of compound E in the form of its acetate. Soon there was a second request for 2 grams. These amounts could be prepared without difficulty, but as the requests increased, both in quantity and frequency, the scale of work was enlarged. Without describing the chemical research required, it is obvious that when a process of manufacture is enlarged to a scale ten, twenty, or forty times the original, an unbelievable amount of costly work must be carried out.

The Department of Research and Development of Merck and Co. provided an uninterrupted supply of compound E. It was the only source for this hormone that was used for the initial stages of the investigation carried out at the Mayo Clinic.

My laboratory at the Mayo Foundation was a necessary link between Merck and Co. and St. Mary's Hospital. Successful use of compound E by the clinician depended on a constant supply of the "free" hormone suspended as a fine powder in a sterile isotonic solution of sodium chloride. From the beginning of project "rheumatoid arthritis" I assumed this responsibility. The procedure had six aspects: procurement, removal of the acetate group, pulverization, size of particles, sterility, and purity of the hormone.

Procurement of the acetate of compound E from Merck and Co. proceeded without incident except on two occasions when it was necessary to have a rush order sent by air by special arrangement with a pilot of Northwest Airlines. I met the plane at 10:00 P.M., returned to the laboratory, and prepared a solution of the E acetate for removal of the acetate group. The telephone and the cooperation of the pilot permitted the schedule to be maintained without interruption. Although the total supply equaled the total amount required during the first few months, we could not build up a reserve of "free" compound E that could be used for experimental purposes.

We were carrying on an enterprise on a shoestring. The businessman can overdraw his bank account with no serious consequences, but in our venture an overdraft meant that some patient could not receive compound E for a day or more. Somehow we managed to meet each deadline. The frenzy and anxiety were all in the day's work, but sometimes I felt that there should be a column on the patient's chart for the record of the worry, frustration, and anxiety of those who served but were unseen.

Removal of the acetate group was considered necessary because the acetate of compound E was insoluble. The physiologic effect of the hormone was dependent upon the rate of absorption. If we had injected compound E acetate in the form of coarse crystals it would have been absorbed so slowly that convincing clinical results could not have been obtained.

Pulverization of "free" compound E was achieved at first by use of mortar and pestle. After the first few grams of compound E had been thus prepared, I realized the inconvenience and risk associated with this method. The mortar, pestle, and isotonic solution of sodium chloride were sterilized by heat, and the hormone was sterilized by crystallization from alcohol, but the mortar was open to the atmosphere, and sterilization of the hand that held the pestle was questionable. It was imperative that all the particles pass through the needle of the syringe, and it was desirable to have the powder so fine that it would not settle rapidly out of suspension. The only safe procedure was to grind the powder for a long time. This, however, increased the risk of contamination.

I decided to modify this step, but consultation of catalogues and letters of inquiry soon disclosed the fact that no ready-made apparatus was available. The problem had been solved in respect to the grinding of material in quantities of the order of pounds or even tons, but nothing could be found to grind minutely material that weighed a few grams.

One incident lingers in my mind. Grinding of a suspension of compound E with glass beads rotated in a small, flat-bottomed flask had not been satisfactory. I substituted steel ball bearings for the glass beads and started rotating the flask containing the compound E that would be required within a few days. The next day (a Saturday) I went to the laboratory to separate the steel balls and place the suspended E in a sterile bottle. To my surprise and dismay, I found that the steel balls had given off iron, which, as iron hydroxide, was sufficient to color the entire suspension a chocolate-brown.

Balls of an alloy of steel and nickel were better, but not satisfactory. I was about to send off a rush order for ball bearings made of tungsten carbide. This material is the hardest substance as well as

129

the most expensive for the particular purpose. Before these balls could arrive, we modified the shape of the flask and again tried glass beads. The arrangement was satisfactory.

The size of the particles was obviously important, but I did not realize how important until the matter was demonstrated by autoclaving the suspended solution. It was satisfactory to grind compound E in a mortar, but the size of the particles was much coarser and less uniform than when compound E was pulverized with glass beads by rotating in a glass flask for 18 hours.

Sterility of each bottle of 50 milliliters was tested as routine. This required a minimum of 36 hours. The importance of sterility was obvious, and although all the operations were carried out in a chemical laboratory, great care was exercised. Nevertheless, I did not wish to take all responsibility or to avoid even a discussion of the subject.

On October 23 it was necessary for me to go to a meeting in New York City. About eight days would be required for the trip. I prepared four bottles, a supply of compound E sufficient to treat the three patients who were under observation. This seemed a good time to bring up the matter of sterility. I consulted Dr. T. B. Magath of the Section of Clinical Pathology and received a clear answer. He pointed out that if one of the patients became infected from an injection of compound E, the Mayo Clinic would be liable to a law suit. The method that had been employed was not safe. The standard methods for sterilization—boiling on three successive days or autoclaving—would have to be used.

This advice was sound and conservative. I decided to autoclave the bottles before I left for New York City. This was done with confidence and a certain degree of relief. When I returned, Dr. Slocumb greeted me with the information that something was very much wrong. The condition of all three patients had regressed after they had received the suspension that had been autoclaved. This was true subjectively and objectively. During my absence Dr. Slocumb had taken the autoclaved bottles to Dr. Mason. He had filtered out the suspension of compound E, reground it in a mortar, and resuspended it in salt solution. When the three patients were given the new suspension they all responded without delay.

At the time this phenomenon remained a mystery. The most probable explanation is that when the suspension of compound E was autoclaved the small particles became smaller and the large particles larger. But the result was that they became dense, unbroken crystals. The rate at which they were dissolved was not sufficient to produce a favorable influence. Since the same material was effective after re-grinding, it follows that the compound E had not been destroyed by autoclaving.

After this demonstration we were forced to return to pulverizing the compound with glass beads. I am proud of the record that was made. More than 1500 injections were given without one incident of infection.

Purity of the hormone was taken for granted. Analysis of the compound E prepared in my laboratory showed that the material was of the highest purity. After we had devised a satisfactory method for the clinical use of E, we examined a sample and discovered an impurity. The new compound was recognized without difficulty. It was closely related to compound E and was made during the last step in the preparation of the hormone. This step was the introduction of the double bond in ring A of compound E. The new compound had the same structure, but, in addition, a second double bond was present in ring B. It will be designated $\Delta 6$. It was readily shown that when compound E was produced on a small scale, very little of the $\Delta 6$ compound was formed, but when compound E was made on a large scale, as much as 3 percent could be $\Delta 6$.

These were interesting chemical facts, but at the time we were concerned about the influence of $\Delta 6$ on rheumatoid arthritis. Months later we showed that the $\Delta 6$ was not toxic and that it exerted less than half the effect of E. However, when $\Delta 6$ was first discovered as an impurity in E, our chief desire was to remove it. Again we believed that we faced an emergency. The problem was to devise a method to purify E, but the only E with which to work was needed for treatment of patients. A simple method was soon found and the emergency passed. This was the last obstacle encountered in the development of a method for the use of compound E as a therapeutic agent.

For the members of my laboratory there were many other problems, but the clinical results were a constant source of encouragement and reward. We had given our answer to the question, "What must be done to establish the value of compound E in clinical medicine?"

We had devised a method for application of the hormone as a new tool.

During the fall of 1948 the administrative committee of the Board of Governors of the Mayo Clinic was faced with a decision. Investigation of the chemical nature of the adrenal cortex had been carried on in the laboratory of the Mayo Foundation for eighteen years. I was in my sixty-second year. Was it probable that anything of importance could come from research on the hormones of the adrenal cortex within the remaining three years before my retirement? The situation closely resembled the one that confronted the executive committee of Merck. The time for decision had arrived, but before any decision could be carried out the report of the treatment of Mrs. G. came to the attention of the Board of Governors. The effect of compound E on rheumatoid arthritis was something new and unanticipated. If it could be confirmed, the Board of Governors wished to be of help. If it could not be confirmed, the time for final action had come.

The observations on patients 2, 3, and 4 brought matters to a head. Patient 4 was a member of the Mayo Clinic. His condition had been recorded for several years, and there was the additional advantage that he could express his subjective reactions in medical terms. His response to the administration of compound E had been excellent, and he was fully appreciative. All who saw him were enthusiastic.

It would be possible to continue this type of investigation and to secure a series of cases similar to the first four; however, it seemed wise to make the demonstration on patient 5 as convincing as possible. The Board of Governors appointed a committee to arrange a formal procedure with a placebo and a "blind test." The "adrenal committee" consisted of three clinicians and two chemists. The late Dr. Mandred W. Comfort was chairman, and the other members were Dr. Randolph G. Sprague, Dr. Charles H. Slocumb, Dr. Harold M. Mason, and myself. I was well pleased with this opportunity to apply a crucial test. If patient 5 responded satisfactorily, much would be gained from this formal action of the committee. If the response of patient 5 was not favorable, the sooner we found this out the better it would be for all concerned. Nothing could be gained by postponement and no limitations were to be placed on the severity of the test.

Dr. Comfort asked me to prepare a suspension of some substance that would resemble the suspension of compound E so closely that the two could not be distinguished by inspection. I chose cholesterol. After this had been pulverized with the aid of a detergent, it was not possible to distinguish bottles containing compound E from those containing the placebo. The bottles, numbered consecutively, were given to Dr. Sprague. Only he and I knew which numbers designated compound E. The physician who gave the injections did not know which substance he was giving, and the patient did not know what he was receiving. The clinicians examined the patient daily and made notations, but they did not know what the patient received.

All the individual contemplations, all the conferences and research, all the decisions and action that have been described were directed toward a single objective: a patient. It is always possible that a creative work in chemistry may provide a new and effective agent in the field of clinical medicine, but in such a study the ultimate criterion that guides the physician is a patient. In this case the criterion was a patient in St. Mary's Hospital. Some research in clinical medicine in the past has appeared trustworthy, but time has wasted away all traces of value. Clinical study of new products in rheumatoid arthritis has a record that carries a warning. There are two aspects that make such investigations hazardous. One is selection of suitable patients; the other is evaluation of results.

I am on firm ground when I say that my clinical colleagues were unsurpassed in their ability to select suitable patients and to interpret clinical results. I was glad to cooperate in discussions of physiologic problems and the preparation of compound E. I was relieved to know that in the field of clinical medicine final judgment would be passed by the physicians on the committee.

Administration of compound E to patient number 1 was a probe into a dark area with a new and untried tool. The "blind test" on patient number 5 was designed to be a critical survey of the adrenal cortical hormone, compound E. The last of the crucial moments had arrived. I was confident that the patient would respond in some de-

133

gree, but there could be no assurance that this result would impress the members of the committee and through them the Board of Governors of the Mayo Clinic.

After the bottles for the test had been delivered to Dr. Sprague, I turned to work in the laboratory as the most satisfactory way to pass the time until the committee was ready to report. Patient 5 was placed in the "metabolic unit" on November 28. When he would receive compound E was known only by Dr. Sprague; when or whether he would respond was known to no one.

In December 1948 the weather was mild. Mrs. Kendall had been ill and it was our custom to take a ride in our automobile whenever possible. We returned from such a ride on Christmas afternoon at about 4:00 P.M. It had been a beautiful day and I had enjoyed a mood that was compounded of a deep personal satisfaction and thankfulness that project E already had produced substantial results. The telephone rang. Dr. Hench had called to give this message: "Miracle number 5 has happened at St. Mary's Hospital."

The full story was this:

Patient 5 was the owner of several trucks and carried on a business in transportation. He had come to the clinic because of severe pains in joints and muscles. The diagnosis was rheumatoid arthritis. Aspirin had relieved the pain to some extent, but he was unable to do any work. In St. Mary's Hospital he had books and magazines, but they did not interest him; he could not attend to matters related to his business. He was a miserable victim of a relentless disease.

When patient 5 was placed in the "metabolic unit" it did not seem wise to withhold aspirin. For study in the "metabolic unit" 6 days was one period. The first 18 days of December were passed without injections of either E or the placebo. During the following period patient 5 received injections of cholesterol. These 6 days ended on December 23. The physicians on the committee were unanimous in their conclusions: The condition of patient 5 had not changed in any significant way during the 6 days he had received a daily injection. On December 24 the first injection of compound E was given. He received the second injection of compound E on December 25, and during that Christmas day the miracle happened. Patient 5 was relieved of pain; he left his bed and walked up and down the corridor and up and down a flight of stairs. He became interested in the reading matter in his room and began to think seriously about his business.

The elaborate precautions and meticulous care exercised in the treatment of patient 5 permitted all members of the committee to express their opinions without reservation. The consensus was that the adrenocortical hormone, compound E, exercises a favorable influence on the symptoms of rheumatoid arthritis. One member expressed it, "I capitulate."

The result of this test was so dramatic and convincing that after December 25, 1948, no one could challenge the statement that compound E suppresses the symptoms of rheumatoid arthritis. The "adrenal committee" was not asked to carry out more experiments, but the placebo, cholesterol, was given to other patients to show the length of time that compound E would continue to act after administration of the hormone had been stopped. The patient was unaware of the fact that a placebo was being given, but in every case the condition of the patient clearly indicated which compound had been injected. Project "rheumatoid arthritis" had survived three months of critical scrutiny. It had reached the end of the beginning and was on high ground. New prospects and new objectives became apparent, but now they could be contemplated with confidence.

Dr. Hench had returned to active service at the Mayo Clinic just in time to witness the successful demonstration provided by patient 5. He immediately made plans for a continuation of the study of compound E. During the next three months eighteen more patients received compound E or other hormones of the adrenal cortex. Of these patients not one failed to respond.

Dr. Sprague studied the effect of compound F, which is closely related to E, and made careful observations on a patient in the metabolic unit. The sample of compound F had been isolated from the adrenal cortex in my laboratory.

Through the courtesy of the Upjohn Company the effect of the whole extract of the adrenal cortex was investigated. Each of these projects gave the results that were predicted, but in February an interesting and controversial question was asked. This had to do with the pituitary hormone that stimulates the activity of the adrenal cortex. It was known that the adrenocorticotropic hormone, ACTH, would cause the adrenal cortex to enlarge and to pour its secretion into the blood stream. Since compounds E and F relieved the symptoms of rheumatoid arthritis, administration of ACTH would also be expected to produce a favorable effect. By itself, ACTH would not have any influence, but the hormones of the adrenal cortex released by ACTH should be as effective as they were after separation in crystalline form.

The only reason for expecting that administration of ACTH might have another effect came from the hypothesis advanced by Dr. Hans Selye. For many years Selye had predicted that overactivity of the adrenal cortex is an etiologic factor in a large number of diseases. Among these diseases was rheumatoid arthritis. According to his prediction, the administration of ACTH would not relieve the symptoms of rheumatoid arthritis; rather, it would cause an exacerbation of symptoms.

The Armour Laboratories of Chicago kindly gave us a generous supply of ACTH. When the time came for injections of the pituitary hormone we were guided by the same reasoning that led to the use of 100 milligrams of compound E for a daily dose. It was imperative to show that ACTH would influence the symptoms. The optimal dose could be established at any time.

A dose of 100 milligrams of ACTH was injected into patient 6. The answer was obtained within 3 days: ACTH exerted just as beneficial an effect on rheumatoid arthritis as had compounds E or F.

In January 1949 Merck and Co. assumed responsibility for preparation of the suspension of compound E in isotonic solution of sodium chloride. Throughout a long period of testing I had refined the method of pulverization of compound E to the point at which any insoluble organic substance could be reduced to a fine uniform powder. We had reached the stage at which we could afford to explore the factors that influenced the physiologic response to compound E. The first question concerned the rate of absorption of free compound E, compared with that of E acetate. One of the three major decisions made at the beginning of project "rheumatoid arthritis" was to use the "free" hormone itself—not an ester. Even in the "free" form, the size of the particle was of first importance. Now it seemed possible that if the material was reduced to a very fine powder, the acetate ester could be used. This would save much labor, and in addition four patients could be treated for every three who were given the "free" E.

A suspension of E acetate was ground as fine as possible, and this was substituted for the suspension of "free" E in a series of patients. There was a slight reduction in their response, but this reduction soon passed off, and the activity of E acetate was so satisfactory that after January 1949 use of the "free" hormone was discontinued.

Subsequently, it was shown that compound E or its acetate ester can be given by mouth. This was most important, for it provided a method for administration that could be carried out in the home without the need for a physician or nurse.

Perhaps a critic would remark that we had overlooked the simplest answer to the problem of administering the cortical hormone and had learned the hard way. However, we had no regrets. Each step was planned and the results were firmly established before we contemplated simplification or change. The hard way, under the circumstances, was the safest and surest way.

Thirteen

Compound E Becomes Cortisone

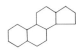

EARLY IN 1949 it became evident that within a few months we would be in a position to make an important announcement in the field of clinical medicine. At a conference with the Board of Governors of the Mayo Clinic it was decided to withhold mention of the influence of compound E on rheumatoid arthritis until just before the annual meeting of the Association of American Physicians. The first presentation of the work would be made before that national organization during the first week of May, but in the latter part of April an initial report would be given at a regular staff meeting of the Mayo Clinic. After these meetings, papers would be read before the American Medical Association and in June at the International Congress of Rheumatologists in New York City.

Every effort was made to prevent the divulging of information about the series of patients who were under treatment, but it was impossible to maintain secrecy. Of one thing we could be sure: no one else had on hand even a small amount of compound E. Merck and Co. had consigned their entire output of this hormone to the Mayo Clinic.

In April 1949, Merck and Co. accepted full responsibility for the preparation of E acetate in the form of a sterile suspension ready for injection. For me this was a welcome release from the obligation I had assumed six months previously.

Throughout the first four months of 1949 clinical investigation of the effects of compound E was expanded. The paper to be presented before the Association of American Physicians was scheduled for May 3, 1949; April 20 was fixed for the first announcement at a meeting of the staff of the Mayo Clinic.

These steps denoted steady progress toward the culmination of project E, but an event early in April marked the beginning of what may be called "fruits of research." Through Dr. T. B. Magath I received a communication from the Board of Governors of the Mayo Clinic which modified profoundly the two years that remained before my retirement. I was asked whether I would like to move into a new laboratory built especially for research in the field of steroids.

My immediate reaction to the question was an unqualified yes, but many facets of the problem became apparent and final acceptance came only after much deliberation. There were two aspects that required consideration: "pure research" in steroid chemistry and an adequate and uninterrupted source of compound E for use in the Mayo Clinic.

For all the uncertainties there was one answer that was satisfactory: compound E could be made on whatever scale was desirable. I believed that production of compound E for clinical use in Rochester was adequate justification for creation of the new laboratory. In addition, enlarging the scope of pure research was a stimulating challenge. I did not regard the new unit as a gamble. Rather, it afforded an opportunity and was a reward for the success that good fortune had brought to us.

As soon as my answer was conveyed to the Board of Governors, they approved the project, plans were drawn as fast as possible, and work was started without delay.

A short time before the announcement of the clinical results on April 20 an incident occurred which, although trifling, was of interest to the rheumatologists at the clinic. A group of prominent rheumatologists who were in Rochester gathered in Dr. Hench's house. They knew that a new chapter on rheumatoid arthritis was being written, but none of them knew the nature of the product that was being used. As each one entered the house he was given a slip of paper and was asked to write his guess concerning the nature of the material. The guesses were distributed over a wide range, but "hormones of the adrenal cortex" did not appear on a single slip. This was a reassurance that no one would make a statement that would precede our own, but there was always the possibility that someone would come upon an observation that would arouse his interest in the adrenal cortex.

One such paper did appear, in *Science,* March 18, 1949, by Leon Hellman. It was concerned with ACTH and gout. Since ACTH exerts an influence on gout and since the effect of ACTH is mediated solely through the adrenal cortex, we realized that this gland would soon be brought under study. However, not much progress could be achieved before our results were made public.

Seven months after the first injection of compound E in a patient with rheumatoid arthritis, we were prepared to announce the clinical results. Regardless of how many times the paper would be repeated subsequently, or how distinguished the audience might be, the "first night" bore a special significance for Dr. Hench and myself.

It was a memorable meeting. Every member of the staff of the Mayo Clinic and Mayo Foundation who could be there was present. Every seat in Plummer Hall was taken, and chairs were placed in the aisles, but many sat on the window sills and even around the platform. Others stood along the sides of the hall and even out to the elevators. Everyone was filled with anticipation and enthusiasm. Seldom has an advance in clinical medicine been made known under more auspicious circumstances.

Twenty-three patients had received a series of injections of compound E. Motion pictures had been made before and after the use of the hormone in each case, and quotations of statements about subjective changes were available.

Dr. Hench emphasized that we were not reporting a cure or even a possible treatment of rheumatoid arthritis. Rather, we wished to present the use of a new tool that now could be employed for a study of the physiologic and pharmacologic influence of the adrenal cortex. He gave a brief review of the history of rheumatoid arthritis and of his own contributions in regard to the effects of jaundice, pregnancy, and the reversibility of the disease. He pointed out the possibility that reversal of symptoms might be brought about by "substance X." Was "substance X" a hormone of the adrenal cortex?

After Dr. Hench presented his paper, the motion-picture film

141

was shown. This illustrated the remarkable changes that had occurred in some of the patients. Only a phlegmatic person can watch that film without a lump in his throat or a mist over his eyes. For those who had known and worked with the patients it was a source of deep emotion.

As I walked to the speaker's desk after these two superlative presentations I had a strong inclination to say simply that anything that I could add would be an anticlimax, and sit down. Then I realized that everything that had been accomplished had been made possible by the long years of patient research on the chemistry of the cortical hormones. As the spokesman for all who had devoted many years to this problem, I was determined to make it clear that "pure research" in biochemistry sometimes can supply a vital link for use by the clinician.

How well I succeeded I do not know, but the applause that broke loose immediately after the conclusion of the program has never been equaled at any other meeting that I have attended.

The applause was not confined to Plummer Hall. The next morning a visiting physician who had been present came to my office to add his congratulations. He then insisted that compound E would surely be of value in the treatment of certain forms of nephritis. Time has shown that he was right.

Before noon on that same day I received a telephone call from Denver, Colorado. The director of research at E. R. Squibb and Sons called to say that that company wanted to give the Mayo Clinic a grant of $5,000.

Dr. Fordyce R. Heilman of the Mayo Clinic remarked, "You are going to be on the receiving end for some time."

The chairman of the Board of Governors wrote me a note that I shall always cherish.

Dr. Donald C. Balfour, who was familiar with many of the dark days in the past, was well pleased and said so in a note.

These are samples of the post-announcement reactions. It was good to be alive, but when one thought of the ravages of rheumatoid arthritis it was not possible to be satisfied or conceited. The dominant reaction was one of humility. We had made a beginning; we were far from making a conclusion.

The time allotted for presentation of the paper before the Association of American Physicians was limited to twelve minutes. This required deletion of much that had been given on April 20, but the film was so convincing that little more was needed. As at the staff meeting, the hall was crowded and the audience was keenly interested. The discussion and applause showed the approval of the auditors. This was a national society; the press was well represented at the meeting. Compound E, a hormone of the adrenal cortex, had moved front and center stage and stood in the spotlight.

Publicity concerning compound E had been anticipated, and an agreement between the Mayo Clinic and the department of public relations of Merck and Co. had been made. This agreement was followed in every detail, but beyond this the Mayo Clinic could not go. As the interest of the public increased, it was inevitable that the opportunity would be used to push other products as far as possible into the spotlight beside compound E. At least one company that sold vitamin E initiated an advertising campaign for the use of vitamin E in arthritis.

The name compound E was laboratory jargon, and since it seemed certain that the hormone some day would be included in the Pharmacopoeia, a distinctive name needed to be selected for the compound.

Dr. Hench came to my laboratory one day in May, 1949, and made the suggestion that the time had come for us to start looking for a name. I promised to think it over and the next day I was prepared. My thoughts had been aided by a process of elimination. The chemical name of compound E is 17-hydroxy-11-dehydrocorticosterone. Since the name should contain not more than two or three syllables, it was reduced to "corticosterone." Removal of "ticoster" left "corsone." Dr. Hench made the point that in "corsone" the stress fell on the syllable "cor," which implied action on the heart. He added the letters "ti" and the word "cortisone" was coined.

The name cortisone was launched on its career at the Seventh International Congress of Rheumatologists in the ballroom of the Waldorf-Astoria Hotel in New York City on June 1, 1949. The papers presented by Dr. Hench and myself were essentially the same as those given on April 20. Again the hall was crowded, interest was at a high pitch, and the work was well received.

The word cortisone appeared more and more frequently in the

medical and lay press. The intimate relationship between ACTH and the hormones of the adrenal cortex increased the general interest, and the demand for cortisone and ACTH steadily increased until it seemed insatiable.

During the second half of 1949 Merck and Co. found themselves in an unusual situation. They alone had developed and possessed the know-how for the commercial manufacture of the hormone. The demand for cortisone was reckoned in millions of dollars. The supply was recorded in grams. Some mechanism was required for distribution of the small quantities of the material as they became available. Fortunately the manufacture and distribution of penicillin established an excellent precedent. Following this pattern, Dr. A. N. Richards, president of the National Academy of Sciences, was asked by Merck and Co. to form a committee that would have complete control over the distribution of cortisone. Dr. Chester Keefer of Boston was the chairman; the other members were Drs. Edward A. Doisy, Hans T. Clarke, Cyril N. H. Long, Robert F. Loeb, Eli K. Marshall, and Joseph T. Wearn. This was a satisfactory solution of a problem that could have been a source of bitterness and criticism for many months.

Five parties were involved in patents pertaining to the manufacture of cortisone: Merck and Co., Ciba and Co., Organon, the Schering Corporation, and the Mayo Clinic. Only those held by Merck and Co. and the Mayo Clinic covered the manufacture of cortisone. The others had been issued some years earlier and applied only in a general way. One prohibited the use, except to the patent owner, of any steroid that had a ketone group at carbon 11 and an atom of bromine at carbon 12. Nevertheless, the three other companies held the patents, and if they chose to do so they could block the manufacture and sale of cortisone by Merck and Co. It was necessary to make some working arrangement, and this had to be done without delay.

What was needed was an independent party to bring the five into agreement. This situation was one ready-made for the Research Corporation of New York. Representatives of this body were asked to serve, and in a short time conflict and confusion were replaced with goodwill and harmony.

One desire was held in common by all the manufacturing companies: none of them wished to have a monopoly on the sale of cortisone; all of them wanted to have the approval of the U.S. Department of Justice for any agreement that was made.

The Research Corporation was given authority to grant licenses to each of the four manufacturing companies originally concerned and to any other company that complied with the terms of the agreement. Each of the contracting parties could use any of the patents held by the other members of the group. A small royalty was collected from each member that sold cortisone, and this was distributed among all members of the agreement.

Acceptance of these terms removed all interference with the manufacture and sale of cortisone. The Research Corporation had performed a great and lasting service.

Patents are issued only to those who make the invention, but in many cases a patent is owned by the company or institution that supported the work and provided the necessary capital. Patents were granted to me and other members of the laboratory as each new step in the preparation of cortisone was devised. The Mayo Clinic did not propose to exploit these patents for financial gain. Yet the Mayo Clinic did wish to be in a position to prevent any use of the scientific contributions made by members of its staff that would be contrary to the principles of the Mayo Clinic and of the medical profession. As soon as the agreement had been prepared, I assigned all my interest in the patents to the Mayo Clinic, which in turn gave them unconditionally to the Research Corporation.

No physician engaged in the practice of medicine should profit from the exploitation of any drug, vaccine, or appliance used in the practice of medicine. This is a time-honored statement; it has been the policy of the Mayo Clinic from its beginning.

The method for isolation of thyroxin was patented, but when the patent was issued, Dr. W. J. Mayo offered it to the board of trustees of the American Medical Association. The gift of the patent was made unconditionally, but Dr. Mayo asked me to assist the lawyer, George Granger, in the draft of the deed of gift. No restrictions were mentioned, but we did include a paragraph to the effect that the board should employ diligence in the commercial development of that hormone. When the document was given to Dr. Mayo he drew a line through all our carefully worded paragraphs and wrote instead, "to do with as they shall see fit."

The incident made a strong impression on me. What was the best policy for the Mayo Clinic in 1920 would still be the best policy in 1950, insofar as it concerned financial return from patents in medical affairs.

It certainly was the best policy for the Mayo Clinic to pass ownership of the cortisone patents to the Research Corporation, but should I also relinquish all financial interest in the future sales of cortisone? The share of the Research Corporation of the royalties from the sale of cortisone certainly would grow to a large sum; why, it might be asked, should I not receive a certain percentage of this? At the time that this question arose, the Mayo Clinic did not have a policy that could be applied. I expressed the belief that no member of the staff should profit from patents issued for work carried out in the laboratories of the Mayo Clinic. After full discussion such a policy was adopted by the Board of Governors.

One consideration assumed prime importance in forming my attitude. The active years of my life had been spent in chemical research at the Mayo Foundation. During the same interval other investigators had carried on research in pathology, physiology, anatomy, bacteriology, parasitology, surgery, clinical chemistry, and biophysics. No one of these scientists could make a contribution in his chosen field that could be patented with results comparable to the opportunities in chemistry. All members of the laboratory group had devoted their lives to science; any policy adopted by the Mayo Clinic should include them all. In the long run teamwork is of more value than solo performances.

I had consulted with, and received invaluable help from, many of those who worked in other disciplines. If I received financial reward, should I divide it among my colleagues? If I did not divide it, would this callous behavior produce bitterness and division?

Perhaps public opinion and medical practice will change in the matter of private gain from patented discoveries, and perhaps present customs will be revised. Until that time, I believe that all scientists in a medical institution should be willing to conform to established policy. I do not regret my choice of action.

146

The year 1949 presented Merck and Co. with problems so important that the well-being of the company was at stake. The clinical reports from the use of cortisone continued to be encouraging, but the outlay of capital for the large-scale production of the hormone was estimated at many millions of dollars. There were questions that could not be answered. Would ACTH prove to be so effective that it would eliminate the use of cortisone? Would some other abundant and cheap member of the steroid family prove to be "just as good"? Would some simple compound, not a steroid, be effective? Would some chemist find a short direct conversion of a bile acid to cortisone and thus eliminate the expensive process currently used for preparation of the hormone? Finally, would some plentiful and cheap source of a suitable steroid other than bile be discovered?

The activity of cortisone in rheumatoid arthritis was so dramatic and the need for the treatment of patients so great that Merck and Co. considered no alternative but to go ahead.

Time has brought answers to all the questions. We now know that the board of directors acted wisely and courageously. We know that cortisone became available first in a trickle and finally in full volume. But only a few chemists know about the heroic struggle in the Department of Research and Development that made this possible. Dr. Max Tishler directed the work; his quiet but effective leadership has since been recognized with many honors. Dozens of new chemists were engaged, vacations were postponed or forgotten, overtime was a part of every day, and unfailing devotion to the job was expected of every man.

The conversion of a bile acid to cortisone required more than thirty different reactions. These were divided into three groups, and each group was intensely explored by a different "task force." Instead of starting at the beginning and working through to the end, each group was carried along simultaneously with the others, and the entire operation was kept in focus. This procedure was successful, and the achievement of Dr. Tishler and his associates in the laboratories of Merck and Co. will stand as a landmark in the annals of industrial chemistry.

When Merck and Co., in 1946, decided to proceed with the preparation of compound E, it was impossible to foresee how the

147

hormone would be used in clinical medicine or to know what amount would be required for a clinical investigation of the compound. However, it was necessary to decide what amount should be made to serve as pilot and pathfinder for its preparation from bile acid. For compound A, 5 grams had been chosen as the target, and for compound E this same goal was selected, but because of the extra steps required for E, the weight of starting material was increased to 1269 pounds. However, between mid-1946 and the end of 1949, many steps were much improved. Instead of the anticipated 5 grams, the total yield was 942 grams.

Even this bonanza could not relieve in any degree the pressure on Dr. Tishler and his associates for more and more E, but it did provide sufficient material for the early stages of the examination of the activity of the hormone.

The weeks between March and August, 1949, were one long procession of authentic reports and seemingly incredible rumors about the wondrous cures brought about by the newest miracle drug, cortisone. In Rochester, these resulted in a subtle but obvious change that was not limited to the staff of the Mayo Clinic. The carpenters, plumbers, and painters working on the new laboratory were told about its purpose, and the effect was galvanic. In four months the entire building was transformed. Every laborer wanted to be in on the story, and all gave of their strength and skill with full measure.

The laboratory was ready for occupancy in August, 1949.

There were many reasons why the offer of a new laboratory was accepted with pleasure, gratitude, and satisfaction. In the first place, such a laboratory would be tangible recognition of the contribution made by biochemistry to clinical medicine. It would be devoted to research in the field of steroids and to production of cortisone for clinical use in the Mayo Clinic. As soon as Merck and Co., could increase its rate of production, there would be no good reason for preparation of the hormone in Rochester. But in 1949 the yield of cortisone from bile acid was less than 0.5 percent, and the demand increased with each new article about the hormone in the lay and medical press. The question of when supply and demand would be brought into balance could not be answered.

While construction was under way members of the new staff were assembled. The group was strengthened by the return of Dr.

H. L. Mason, whose experience in the field of steroids afforded theoretical help and wise counsel. Our receptionist was Miss Helen M. Cassidy, who also could take the most technical dictation without a flaw, and type more pages per day and with fewer mistakes than any secretary we ever had. Her skill and gracious manner won my lasting appreciation. In April 1950 Warren F. McGuckin returned after an absence of more than five years. He had meanwhile acquired the degree of doctor of philosophy. Much of the credit for the manufacture of cortisone in the new plant goes to him. Bernard F. McKenzie and Gene Worock were responsible for the first steps. Vernon Mattox, Frank Colton, and William R. Nes made important contributions in research. Several papers of first quality were written and intensive research in the steroid field was carried out in the years 1949 and 1950. We were in a position to make a series of observations that brought credit and prestige to the laboratory.

Outside the laboratory David Van Dorp will be remembered for many well-fought games of chess; H. R. (Gerry) Nace for the hours he spent fishing long after sunset; Warner Florsheim for his optimism, thoughtfulness, and persistence; Timothy O'Connor for his ever-ready Irish wit and cheerfulness. On one mid-winter morning with the temperature between −20 and −30 degrees F., O'Connor arrived at the laboratory, wearing his clothes over his pajamas and a scarf wound over—not around—his head, with hat perched on top of the scarf. He never had experienced such cold in Ireland.

In the 1940s Dr. Weyer of the Research Corporation told me about finding a small black box in a drawer of a little-used desk. It contained the one-millionth dollar paid by Merck and Co. in royalties for the license to manufacture vitamin B1. The incident remained in my mind, and when Merck started commercial production of cortisone in 1949 I asked them to give me a small sample of the millionth gram of the hormone. I expected to wait four or five years, but in May 1951 I received the sample, beautifully mounted in a block of lucite. Beside it there was a sample of the first gram of cortisone given to a patient.

Stated in familiar terms, one million grams of cortisone is more than a ton. This gives an idea of the magnitude of research and effort required for this amazing achievement.

"The announcement in 1949 of cortisone's dramatic effectiveness in treating rheumatoid arthritis touched off one of the greatest bursts of excitement in the entire history of drug therapy." Cortisone was acclaimed "one of the most significant discoveries of our generation." It was hailed as being "among the biggest advances that medicine has ever made in a single leap. . . . In the wake of the stupendous publicity given cortisone in treating rheumatoid arthritis, the clamor for the new 'miracle drug' reached almost hysterical proportions."

These quotations are from "Arthritis and Arthritis Drugs" by Howard J. Sanders.* The statements were made before it was recognized that cortisone and its derivatives are a two-edged sword. When they are administered in large doses over long periods of time, symptoms of hypercortisonism appear. The effective use of cortisone was retarded by intemperate criticism that was highly emotional and unscientific.

As the years have passed a more reasonable attitude has displaced both extreme praise and bitter denunciation. The late Dr. Joseph J. Bunim has pointed out that in addition to the three diseases first studied (rheumatoid arthritis, rheumatic fever, and systemic lupus erythematosus), cortisone and its derivatives are now used in certain diseases of the eye, skin, kidneys, lungs, heart, blood, blood vessels, gastrointestinal tract, connective tissue, and muscle, and that in general the cortico-steroids have been found effective in suppressing reactions of inflammation and hypersensitivity.

* *Chemical Engineering News,* August 12, 1968, 46–73.

Fourteen

Nobel Prize

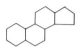

ON A MORNING in late October 1922, Professor and Mrs. Archibald V. Hill were eating breakfast in their home in London. Mrs. Hill picked up the morning paper and began to read. Presently she looked up and asked, "Who do you think won the Nobel Prize in Medicine and Physiology?" Professor Hill mentioned two eminent British physiologists. "No," Mrs. Hill replied, "you did."

In the afternoon of a day in late October 1937, Mrs. Albert Szent-Györgyi in Szeged, Hungary, received a telephone call informing her that her husband had been awarded the Nobel Prize in Medicine and Physiology. During the evening the official message was received.

These are but two instances of an event that has occurred annually since 1900. By 1950 the custom of making the first announcement of the awards of Nobel Prizes to the recipients had been practiced and perfected to a high degree of smoothness and credibility. The American correspondents of Swedish newspapers, especially, vied with one another to be the first to convey the information.

On the evening of October 25, 1950, one correspondent could wait no longer. Although the vote of the faculty that selected the recipients in Medicine and Physiology would not be taken until the following day, he telephoned my married daughter who lived in western New York State. He warned her not to tell anyone about the

151

phone call because the selection was not yet official, but he had no doubt that the Nobel Prize in Medicine and Physiology would be awarded to me. He wanted to know something about me. What were my likes and dislikes? Did I enjoy sports? Was I a member of a church or club?

As soon as she could recover from the surprise, she telephoned her brother in nearby Rochester, New York. She explained that she was not to mention the award of the Nobel Prize and then she asked, "What shall I do?" The answer was short. "For God's sake hurry up and telephone your father."

The following morning I had an appointment with the dentist and left word with my secretary where I could be reached. At 10:30 A.M. I was called to the telephone. The message came from one of the Swedish newspaper correspondents but again it was made clear that the vote had not been taken.

I went home for lunch. At 11:45 A.M. the telephone rang and I listened once more to the now familiar message. When the speaker reached the point of warning me not to mention the conversation, I interrupted and asked him not to call me again until the vote had been taken and the outcome was officially announced. At 1:30 P.M. on October 26, the official announcement was made. The Nobel Prize in Medicine and Physiology for 1950 was awarded to Edward C. Kendall, Philip S. Hench, and Tadeus Reichstein for their investigations of the hormones of the adrenal cortex. Both the medical profession and the reading public were eager to know the latest news about cortisone, and the award of the Nobel Prize brought a flood of personal congratulations, telephone calls, telegrams, and letters from associates, friends, and strangers.

A newspaper correspondent in New York sent congratulations and predicted that other still greater prizes would be awarded in the future. By chance, Nobel laureate Archibald V. Hill was a visitor in Rochester, Minnesota, and I showed him that telegram. He remarked that he could not imagine any greater award based on scientific value.

The American physicist Clinton J. Davisson said, when he received the Nobel Prize, that a recipient is transformed "overnight from an exceedingly private citizen to something in the nature of a

* *Nobel the Man and His Prizes* (Stockholm, Sohlmans Verlag, 1927), 313.

semi-public institution."* And so it seemed to Mrs. Kendall and me. All our colleagues in the Mayo Foundation and friends in Rochester wanted to show their pleasure and satisfaction. One example was typical and noteworthy. The vice president of the Chicago Northwestern Railroad invited Mrs. Kendall and me to start our trip to Stockholm as guests of the railroad from Rochester to Chicago in the president's private car. On the day of departure the car was brought to Rochester. A luncheon was served in it to members of the laboratory, and a dinner for twelve of our friends was served before the train left for Chicago. The dinner was a bright, gay, and joyous affair, with something above and beyond an ordinary social gathering. Perhaps it was the realization that the send-off party was not for the Nobel Prize alone. Behind the award was cortisone, and cortisone was available to everyone—not just Nobel laureates.

One more item of that evening deserves mention. At the center of the dinner table a beautiful arrangement of flowers created a "homey atmosphere." However, these flowers were of special significance. Attached to the container was a card with a message. "Best wishes from the railroad employees." That meant the ticket agents, baggage men, and others who wanted to show their interest and good will.

A group of our friends came to the car to say "bon voyage," and after the events of the day we had the feeling of ambassadors with the blessing of everyone. From the lounge in the rear of the car we watched the lights of Rochester recede, and after a short visit with our host we retired to wide beds with four legs—not ordinary Pullman berths. In the morning we were awakened by a buzzer, and at the door stood the waiter with two tall glasses of freshly squeezed orange juice. We finished breakfast as we approached Chicago, we thanked the chef and waiter, expressed our sincere appreciation to our host, and passed into the station. Our fairy-story trip was over. (*Sic transit gloria mundi*. On our return home from Stockholm we planned to take a day train from Chicago to Rochester, but when I tried to purchase two seats in the Pullman chair car I was told that none were available. We went home in the day coach.)

When we began to make plans for the trip to Stockholm we were delighted to learn that we would have as traveling companions our close friends Albert J. Lobb and his wife, Mary. Mr. Lobb was going to the Nobel Festival to represent the Mayo Foundation and the University of Minnesota. He was on the Board of Governors of the former and a member of the Board of Regents of the latter. The Lobbs were at the dinner in the president's car and they had added a good share of the gaiety on that occasion.

The four of us crossed a well-behaved Atlantic Ocean on the steamship *Oslofjord* to Copenhagen and Oslo. Mr. Lobb was a friend of Mrs. Eugenie Anderson, then United States Ambassador to Denmark, and when she learned of our presence in Copenhagen, we were invited to her home for lunch. In Oslo Dr. and Mrs. Per Laland were hosts at a pleasant luncheon in the hotel at the top of Holmenkollen.

Soon after announcement of the Nobel Prize I received a request from Stockholm for a recorded acceptance of the prize that could be broadcast to the people of Sweden. The message was recorded in Rochester and air-mailed to Stockholm, but the death of King Gustav V on October 29 caused the broadcast to be postponed. When we arrived at the railroad station in Stockholm on December 8, I was surprised to hear my name on the public address system: "Dr. Kendall has just arrived and here he is." Then the record made six weeks earlier was played. It sounded as though I were speaking "live" from the railroad station.

From the railroad station we and the Lobbs were taken to the Grand Hotel. To each of the new laureates was assigned an attaché from the Swedish Foreign Office, who served as escort and adviser during our stay in Stockholm. Our sensitive and efficient escort, Bengt Odeval, assumed a serious personal interest in our sojourn and was most helpful.

The year 1950 was the fiftieth anniversary of the award of the Nobel Prize, and the Nobel Festival in December 1950 was of special interest. All former recipients were invited to attend; thirty accepted the invitation, and twenty-six of them were in Stockholm. Among these were four Americans: Dr. Herbert Spencer Gasser, Director of the Rockefeller Institute; Professor Isidor Isaac Rabi, physicist of Columbia University; Professor Percy Williams Bridgman, physicist of Harvard; and Professor Otto Stern, Emeritus Professor of Physics of the Carnegie Institute of Technology. English Nobel laureates Baron Adrian of Cambridge, Sir William Lawrence Bragg, Ernst

Boris Chain, Sir Henry Hallett Dale, Sir Alexander Fleming, Archibald Vivian Hill, and Sir George Paget Thomson were present, as well as Professor Corneille J. F. Heymans from Belgium and Madame Irène Joliot-Curie from France.

The presence of the former recipients enlarged the scope and splendor of the occasion, and the recipients of the 1950 awards appreciated their good fortune in being chosen in this particular year.

All the new laureates and former recipients occupied rooms in the Grand Hotel. The quietest laureate was William Faulkner, who was not seen to speak to anyone, and the busiest one was Dr. Hench, who was usually surrounded by a group of newsmen eager to learn of the latest clinical results of cortisone. Another reason for Dr. Hench's popularity was the family circle that accompanied him to Stockholm—his mother-in-law, Mrs. John Kahler, his wife, Mary, and four children, Kahler, Mary, Susan, and John.

The first scheduled meeting of the laureates in medicine and physiology was a reception at the Nobel Foundation House on Saturday afternoon, December 9. There we had the opportunity to meet our hosts, His Excellency Dr. Lars Binger Ekeberg and the other officers of the Nobel Foundation. Following the reception, the rector and faculty of the Caroline Institute gave an impressive dinner for the new and former laureates in medicine and physiology who were in Stockholm; diplomatic representatives of several countries, with their wives, were among the guests. This was the first occasion at which a toast was proposed to honor Dr. Hench and me. Professor Reichstein had planned to be present but was delayed by fog and did not arrive until Sunday afternoon.

Dr. Hench and I responded to the toast. I said only a few words. After the dinner the wife of the British ambassador, in congratulating me, said that mine was the shortest speech she had ever heard.

The scheduled program for Sunday, December 10, was long and arduous. In the morning the new and old Nobel laureates were taken to the nearby cemetery for a short ceremony during which a wreath was placed on the grave of Nobel. The temperature was well above the melting point, and the snowfall of Saturday night was soft and slushy. Above Nobel's grave some pine trees with long needles were heavily laden with a blanket of snow. As we stood with hats off, a water-soaked snowy avalanche fell with a muffled thud, striking the ground between Sir Henry Dale and me. Had it fallen two feet to the right or left it would have covered one or the other of us.

From the meeting at Nobel's grave the new recipients assembled at the Concert Hall to be informed about the ceremony that would be held that afternoon. Our part was short and not complicated. After the rehearsal we returned to the Grand Hotel, ate lunch in our rooms, dressed for the award ceremony, and awaited the arrival of our escort to accompany us to the Concert Hall. This interval was a moment of highest significance. I relived some of the most difficult days in the past and the way problems in the laboratory that were complete roadblocks barred progress until they were overcome. Other memories were of my life with the companion who married me in 1915. I was happy that the award had come when we could share it, for in truth, that was the way we had lived. I was always strongly motivated, but Becky added an incentive to this drive. I wanted to do my best and succeed for her sake. Her life was so fine and self-effacing that she had endeared herself to all who know her. The love and devotion she gave to our four children have been reflected in their lives as they took their place in the world.

Other sobering thoughts concerned the events of the immediate future. Only eleven Americans had been awarded a Nobel Prize in medicine and physiology during the preceding fifty years. Dr. Hench and I wanted to perform our part in the Nobel Festival without fault. The people of Stockholm realize that the annual award of the Nobel Prize is a unique event. The Concert Hall was filled to capacity (about 2,000), extra chairs were placed in the aisles, and 3,500 people watched the ceremony on television screens in two nearby auditoriums.

All who attended the Concert Hall were in formal attire. This was true even of the photographers, of whom there were many. The Nobel Festival of 1950 was a solemn occasion. One was conscious of the continuity of the Nobel Foundation with its chain of awards that reaches back to 1901 and will doubtless continue even longer into the future. December 10, 1950, was a link in that long chain, but it was our day, the high point of our lives, and our emotions were deeply stirred.

In keeping with the solemn Festival was the atmosphere created by the beautiful interior of the Concert Hall, decorated with a profusion of plants and flowers that had been flown to Stockholm from Holland.

During the preceding fifty years Gustav V as crown prince and king had presented most of the prizes to the recipients. The death of this well-loved king six weeks before the Nobel Festival of 1950 caused some modification in the plans. The most obvious change was in the formal black gowns, set off with deep white collars, worn by the ladies of the royal family and others.

Dr. Ekeberg, as Lord High Steward, opened the proceedings with a welcome to the royal family and guests, which was followed by a tribute to the late king and a brief review of the life of Alfred Nobel. Following the address the prizes were conferred. The order in which we were seated was the same as the order of the prizes mentioned in Nobel's will, and this proved to be the order in which the prizes were presented. The ritual was the same for all the prizes. The recipient remained seated while his "sponsor" presented a short review of his work and explained why his contribution was considered worthy of a Nobel Prize. Following this presentation the recipient rose from his chair and received a personal citation from the sponsor. In each case the sponsor closed his remarks with the same formula. "I now have the honor of asking you to accept the Nobel Prize for 1950 from the hand of His Gracious Majesty, the King." Immediately thereafter, the orchestra played a short interlude while the recipient walked to the platform at the front of the stage, bowed to King Gustav VI, turned to the right, and descended a flight of steps to the auditorium floor. As each recipient reached the floor, the king rose from his chair in the center of the front row and advanced to greet him. When they met, each laureate received from the king a diploma and the gold medal enclosed in a tooled leather case. The king and the laureate engaged in a short conversation, the king returned to his chair, and the laureate passed to the flight of steps on the right side of the platform and ascended to the stage. When he reached the stage he turned to face the king, made a second bow, and returned to his seat.

The time required for each recipient to accept the prize from the king was not more than two or three minutes. The audience rose as the recipient left his chair and applauded when he received the prize. The orchestra played while he walked down to meet the king and while he returned to his place.

The sponsors for physics, chemistry, and literature read their reviews and citations, but Professor Göran Liljestrand, sponsor for physiology and medicine, did not refer to notes of any kind. For fifteen minutes he delivered from memory an address that was printed in the program and was in the hands of the entire audience. It was an impressive feat. Not once did he depart from the printed word.

During the processional, after the address by Dr. Ekeberg, and between presentations of the awards by the king, the ceremony was enriched by symphonic music played by the Concert Hall orchestra. As a final contribution, the orchestra accompanied the entire audience as they sang the Swedish National Anthem "Du gamla du fria." This marked the end of the convocation, but the climax of the Festival awaited our arrival at the City Hall.

All visitors to Stockholm agree that the City Hall is a beautiful building and to the laureates of 1950 it seemed superbly fitting for the banquet for almost a thousand invited guests. The great Blue Hall was required to seat the guests, but the high ceilings, wide halls, and broad stairway dispelled any sensation of crowding. The floral and other decorations were varied and colorful.

The laureates and a group of honored guests waited while the other invited guests were shown to their places. A fanfare sounded and the group, acompanied with orchestral music, moved forward to their banquet tables. The new laureates and their wives were at the head table. I sat between the wife of Dr. Ekeberg and Frau Von Laue. Mrs. Kendall's table companion was Prime Minister Tage Erlander.

The service was picturesque. With each course, the waiters marched to music down the marble stairs. The tables were decorated with tall candelabra, flowers, and smaller candleholders. Near the close of the banquet, the hall suddenly was darkened, except for the candles on the table. To an accompaniment by the orchestra a long line of waiters appeared on the balcony, each with a tray carried shoulder high. In addition to the dessert, each tray held a figure made of clear ice that was illuminated by electric lights with small

158

batteries frozen inside the ice. At the head of the procession a captain carried a tray with an ice eagle, wings outstretched.

Two toasts were proposed during the banquet: one for the king, one in memory of Nobel. At intervals during the dinner, brief acceptance speeches by the new laureates were given. The trumpeters would sound a fanfare. Then, after a moment of silence, the next speaker's name was announced. After his name was called, each laureate had to pass from the head table to the broad marble stairway, ascend a few steps to a rostrum on the first landing, turn, and face the assembly.

This requirement was somewhat of an ordeal, but for me there were two sources of relief, neither of which was the result of any plan or foresight of mine. The first was the fact that all of the guests at the banquet knew about cortisone and wanted to hear more. Since I was responding to a desire on their part I could devote all of my attention to what I was doing. All thought of how the message would be received was crowded out of my mind.

The second relief arrived just before it was time for my name to be called. I had written my acceptance speech in Rochester. When we left the Grand Hotel to attend the Nobel Festival, I made sure that it was in the pocket of my dress suit, but when I looked for it after we were seated at the head table I could not find it.

Suddenly a wholly unanticipated challenge rose up before me. I had decided not to trust my memory, and I could not remember more than two words of the short speech. I could not say that I was sorry but I would have to be excused from my acceptance speech; I could not be paged to answer a transatlantic telephone call; I could not swoon and ask for a physician. As the minutes ticked off I became more disturbed. Just as I was resigning myself to the inevitable, I looked in my pocket once more. There was the speech, caught in the folds of the program of the ceremony. I was so relieved that when my name was called I walked to the rostrum with firm step and head held high. My voice did not quaver. I spoke with confidence.

Following the speeches of the eight new laureates, the former recipients were represented by the senior laureate, Von Laue. This part of the program was closed by an association of University students. After their leader had greeted the guests at the banquet, and laureate Powell had made an eloquent response, the audience was entertained with choral singing. The students were assembled on a balcony that overlooked the banquet floor and as a finale they proceeded singing down the broad stairway, marched the length of the banquet hall, and, still singing, made their exit at the far end.

The Nobel Festival of 1950 was brought to an end by a reception in the Gold Room followed by dancing in the Blue Hall. Somewhat after midnight Mrs. Kendall and I retired to the Grand Hotel. It had been a memorable day.

Along with the official notice to the recipients of the Nobel Prize for 1950 had been sent a copy of *Les Prix Nobel en 1947,* a recent edition of this annual publication of the Nobel Foundation. It contained the acceptance speeches and also the lectures by the laureates pertaining to their prize-winning works. Nobel's will stipulated that recipients of the prize in medicine and physiology were to be selected by the faculty of the Caroline Institute. We were asked by that institute to deliver our Nobel lectures on Monday afternoon, December 11. Although such a lecture would require the better part of an hour, it was a compilation of results already recorded and did not involve new research. The order of the presentation was Kendall, Hench, Reichstein, and all the addresses were well received.

These lectures were our last official duties at the Nobel Festival. They were followed by a series of social functions for the new laureates and thir wives. Because of the death of King Gustav V the usual banquet at the king's palace was canceled and a dinner was given by the Nobel family at the Grand Hotel. After the dinner the royal family held a reception at the palace. Earlier that day when I remarked to our escort, Mr. Odeval, that I would wear a soft brown hat in the taxi from the hotel to the king's palace, such a distressed look came over the face of our solicitous attaché that I did not argue. On Monday afternoon, after delivering our lectures at the Caroline Institute, Dr. Hench and I visited a hat store where we each rented a high silk hat. This was the first occasion on which either of us had worn this regalia.

During the reception at the palace, we met the king and queen, Princess Sibylla, Prince Bertil, and Prince Wilhelm. The royal family extended a cordial greeting. Prince Bertil had visited Minnesota, and when we met he promptly asked about the weather in that state. As we were waiting in a large anteroom we were near William Faulkner and his daughter Gill, who confided to Mrs. Kendall that her slippers were killing her.

The program at the Museum was furnished by La Société d'Orchestre Académique de Stockholm, the Academic Choir of Stockholm, and a soprano who sang some lovely Swedish songs. This day was brought to a close by a buffet supper.

The festivities of the final two days in Stockholm included a luncheon for the Kendalls and the Henches at the home of Ambassador and Mrs. Butterworth on December 12, followed by a party in the laboratory of Professor Liljestrand. That evening there was a dinner at the home of Nanna Svartz, professor of medicine at the Caroline Institute. She was a member of the subcommittee that examined the publications on the hormones of the adrenal cortex and reported to the faculty of the institute. The report resulted in the selection of Hench, Reichstein, and myself as recipients of the Nobel Prize. Professor Svartz's husband, Dr. Nils Malmbert, was professor of pediatrics at the institute. The dinner included the Henches, Professor Reichstein and his daughter, the Kendalls, the Lobbs, and many friends of the Malmberts.

December 13 was marked by participation in some of the ceremonies of Sweden's annual Lucia Festival, which commemorates the legendary Roman maiden Saint Lucia and ushers in the Christmas season. On the morning of that day we were awakened about seven o'clock by a knock at our hotel-room door. I opened the door and saw a group of six or eight young ladies in long white gowns. On the head of one was a crown with lighted candles; others had trays with food, cups, saucers, and a coffee urn. The leader spoke in clear English: "Will you please get back in bed?" I did, and while the group of young ladies stood at the foot of my bed singing "Santa Lucia" Mrs. Kendall and I were served coffee and saffron buns. We were photographed, and the group moved on to the next room. At the time of the ceremony I thought it was limited to the Nobel laureates, but later I learned that all guests of the hotel were included.

The day was spent in visits to a hospital for arthritis patients, and to other points of interest in Stockholm. After dinner in the Grand Hotel, the Lobbs and Kendalls said good-by to our friends and took the train for Paris. Again we were just plain American tourists.

In Paris we parted from the Lobbs, who were off to England, while we proceeded to Cherbourg. Our trip home on the *Queen Elizabeth* was smooth and uneventful, enlivened by the company of the Hench family and of new friends.

Carl Anderson of Merck and Co., who had been in Europe on a business trip at the time of the Nobel Festival, was returning to the United States on the *Queen Elizabeth*. He was interested to hear about the Nobel Festival and was surprised to learn that Dr. Hench had a motion-picture film with sound recordings of the ceremony in the Concert Hall and the banquet in the City Hall. These two gentlemen then proceeded to concoct a scheme to surprise me. The following morning I met Mr. Anderson on the deck and he remarked that he had a film of some unexpected results of cortisone. He said that he and Dr. Hench had made arrangements to have the film shown in the theater on the ship and invited Mrs. Kendall and me to see it. At the appointed hour we all came to the theater. Dr. Hench made some noncommittal remarks and said he would present the film to me for a Christmas present. Then the film of the Nobel Festival with fine symphonic music was shown. My surprise was complete; I had not known that the film had been made and I certainly was unaware that Dr. Hench had secured a copy before he left Stockholm. Even Dr. Hench was surprised by the music. In Paris he had visited a film store where the picture had been projected for him, but since the machine did not have a sound track, he had not heard the music before.

Christmas in the homes of our married children in Rochester and Pultneyville, New York, and the train trip to Rochester, Minnesota, brought us home early in January 1951. The return, however, was not an anticlimax. The staff of the Mayo Clinic and the nurses of St. Mary's Hospital, as well as smaller groups, wanted to hear about the trip to Stockholm and to see the film of the festival. We were invited to address a dinner meeting of the American Swedish Society in Minneapolis, and after our talks we showed the film. This group could not only appreciate the picture and the music, but also understand the Swedish dialogue.

On the evening of January 12, our changed status in life was recognized with a reception given by the Mayo Clinic in the Mayo Foundation House. This was a formal affair, attended by about 400 guests. No speeches were delivered but each one was eager to express his own congratulations.

As the guests departed they were asked to sign a guest book. This I cherish, for to read the names is to recall their faces, personalities, and my associations with them. On the first page of the volume is the name Alice Mayo and, immediately below, "Chuck Mayo, same city." I can imagine the twinkle in his eye when he wrote those words. He was the only one who added anything to his signature. But then there was only one Chuck Mayo.

The millionth gram of cortisone commemorated by the sample in the block of lucite has a parallel in the use of the hormone in clinical medicine. Somewhere there must reside the millionth patient whose pain was relieved or whose life was saved through the use of cortisone. I have recorded some of the incidents, the hopes, and the difficulties that were a part of this compound's history. To my many colleagues and myself, the millionth patient will remain a symbol of great satisfaction and humble pride in a white crystalline compound —cortisone.

Honors and Awards
Index

Honors and Awards

Awards

John Scott Prize, City of Philadelphia, 1921

Chandler Medal, Columbia University, 1925

Squibb Award, Endocrine Society, 1945

Lasker Award, Lasker Foundation (with P. S. Hench), 1949

Research Corporation Award, Research Corporation of New York, 1949

Page One Award, New York Newspaper Guild (with P. S. Hench), 1950

John Phillips Memorial Award, American College of Physicians, 1950

Remsen Award, American Chemical Society, Maryland Section, 1950

Edgar F. Smith Award, American Chemical Society, Philadelphia Section, 1950

Research Award, American Pharmaceutical Manufacturers Association, 1950

Passano Award, Passano Foundation (with P. S. Hench), 1950

Medal of Honour, Canadian Pharmaceutical Manufacturers Association, 1950

Nobel Prize, Nobel Foundation (with P. S. Hench and T. Reichstein), 1950

Dr. C. C. Criss Award, Omaha Mutual Insurance Association (with P. S. Hench), 1951

Award of Merit, Masonic Foundation (with P. S. Hench), 1951

Cameron Award, University of Edinburgh (with T. Reichstein), 1951

Heberden Award, Heberden Society of London, 1951

Kober Award, Association of American Physicians, 1952

Alexander Hamilton Medal, Alumni of Columbia College, 1961

Scientific Achievement Award, American Medical Association, 1965

Honorary Degrees (Doctor of Science)

University of Cincinnati, 1922
Western Reserve University, 1950
Williams College, 1950
Yale University, 1950
Columbia University, 1951
National University of Ireland, 1951
Gustavus Adolphus College, 1964

Scientific Societies

Member

American Academy of Arts and Sciences
American Chemical Society
American Philosophical Society
American Physiological Society
American Society of Biological Chemists (President 1925-26)
American Society of Experimental Biology and Medicine
American Society of Experimental Pathology
Association of American Physicians
Endocrine Society (President 1930-31)
National Academy of Sciences
Sigma Xi

Honorary Member

Columbian Society of Endocrinology
Heberden Society, London
Royal Society of Medicine of England
Swedish Society of Endocrinology

Index